THE TYPE 2 DIABETIC COOKBOOK FOR THE NEWLY DIAGNOSED

A beginner's guide to 2000+ days of nourishing and healthy diabetic- friendly recipes, perfect for type 2 diabetes and newly diagnosed, with a 31-day meal plan

Marcos Baron

Table of Contents

COPYRIGHT © 2023

CHAPTER ONE

Understanding Type 2 Diabetes

Introduction to Type 2 Diabetes

Type 2 diabetes is a chronic metabolic disorder characterized by insulin resistance, inadequate insulin production, or both. Unlike type 1 diabetes, which typically develops in childhood or adolescence and is caused by the immune system attacking insulin-producing cells in the pancreas, type 2 diabetes usually occurs in adulthood and is strongly associated with lifestyle factors, such as poor diet, lack of physical activity, and obesity. In this section, we will delve into the basics of type 2 diabetes, its causes, symptoms, and the importance of early detection and diagnosis.

Basics of Type 2 Diabetes: Causes and Symptoms

Type 2 diabetes develops when the body becomes resistant to insulin, a hormone produced by the pancreas that helps regulate blood sugar levels. Insulin resistance occurs when the body's cells fail to respond properly to insulin, leading to elevated blood sugar levels. Over time, the pancreas may also become unable to produce enough insulin to compensate for this resistance, resulting in further increases in blood sugar levels.

The exact causes of type 2 diabetes are complex and multifactorial, involving a combination of genetic, environmental, and lifestyle factors. While genetics plays a significant role in predisposing individuals to type 2 diabetes, lifestyle factors such as poor diet, lack of physical activity, and obesity are major contributors to its development. A diet high in processed foods, sugar, and unhealthy fats, combined with sedentary behavior, can increase the risk of obesity and insulin resistance, ultimately leading to type 2 diabetes.

The symptoms of type 2 diabetes can vary from person to person and may develop gradually over time. Common symptoms include frequent urination, excessive thirst, unexplained weight loss, fatigue, blurred vision, and slow wound healing. However, some individuals with type 2 diabetes may not experience any symptoms at all, especially in the early stages of the disease. As a result, many cases of type 2 diabetes go undiagnosed for years, increasing the risk of complications such as heart disease, stroke, kidney failure, and nerve damage.

Importance of Early Detection and Diagnosis

Early detection and diagnosis of type 2 diabetes are crucial for preventing or delaying the onset of complications and improving long-term outcomes. Regular screening for diabetes is recommended for individuals with risk factors such as obesity, sedentary lifestyle, family history of diabetes, and certain ethnic backgrounds. Diagnostic tests for diabetes include fasting blood sugar test, oral glucose tolerance test, and glycated hemoglobin (HbA1c) test, which measures average blood sugar levels over the past two to three months.

Once diagnosed, type 2 diabetes requires ongoing management and monitoring to keep blood sugar levels within target range and reduce the risk of complications. Treatment typically involves lifestyle modifications such as healthy diet, regular exercise, weight management, and medication as needed. In some cases, insulin therapy may be necessary to control blood sugar levels effectively.

Understanding Blood Sugar Levels and Management

Blood sugar, or glucose, is the primary source of energy for the body's cells and tissues. However, elevated blood sugar levels can damage blood vessels and organs over time, leading to complications such as heart disease, stroke, kidney failure, and nerve damage. Therefore, maintaining optimal blood sugar levels is essential for managing type 2 diabetes and reducing the risk of complications.

The target blood sugar levels for individuals with type 2 diabetes may vary depending on various factors such as age, overall health, and presence of other medical conditions. In general, the American Diabetes Association (ADA) recommends the following targets for most adults with diabetes:

- Fasting blood sugar (before meals): 80-130 mg/dL

- Postprandial blood sugar (after meals): less than 180 mg/dL

Achieving and maintaining these target blood sugar levels requires a combination of lifestyle modifications, medication, and regular monitoring. Self-monitoring of blood sugar levels using a glucose meter allows individuals to track their blood sugar levels throughout the day and make necessary adjustments to their treatment plan.

In addition to monitoring blood sugar levels, managing type 2 diabetes also involves adopting a healthy lifestyle that includes:

- Following a balanced diet rich in fruits, vegetables, whole grains, lean proteins, and healthy fats

- Engaging in regular physical activity such as walking, swimming, cycling, or strength training

- Maintaining a healthy weight through portion control, mindful eating, and regular exercise

- Avoiding smoking and excessive alcohol consumption

- Getting regular check-ups and screenings to monitor for complications and adjust treatment as needed

By effectively managing blood sugar levels and adopting a healthy lifestyle, individuals with type 2 diabetes can reduce the risk of complications and improve their quality of life.

Lifestyle Factors and Diabetes Risk

Role of Diet and Physical Activity in Diabetes Prevention

Diet and physical activity play crucial roles in the prevention and management of type 2 diabetes. A healthy diet that is rich in fruits, vegetables, whole grains, lean proteins, and healthy fats can help control blood sugar levels, promote weight loss, and reduce the risk of complications.

A diet high in processed foods, sugar, and unhealthy fats, on the other hand, can contribute to insulin resistance, obesity, and elevated blood sugar levels, increasing the risk of type 2 diabetes and its complications. Therefore, it is essential to focus on nutrient-dense foods and limit the intake of sugary beverages, refined carbohydrates, and saturated fats.

In addition to following a healthy diet, regular physical activity is also important for diabetes prevention and management. Exercise helps improve insulin sensitivity, lower blood sugar levels, promote weight loss, and reduce the risk of cardiovascular disease. The American Diabetes Association (ADA) recommends at least 150 minutes of moderate-intensity aerobic exercise, such as brisk walking or cycling, per week, along with muscle-strengthening activities on two or more days per week.

Impact of Weight Management on Diabetes Control

Obesity is a significant risk factor for type 2 diabetes, as excess body fat, particularly around the abdomen, can increase insulin resistance and blood sugar levels. Therefore, achieving and maintaining a healthy weight is essential for diabetes prevention and management.

Weight management strategies for individuals with type 2 diabetes include:

- Following a balanced diet that emphasizes portion control, nutrient-dense foods, and mindful eating

- Engaging in regular physical activity to burn calories, improve insulin sensitivity, and promote weight loss

- Setting realistic goals for weight loss and tracking progress over time

- Seeking support from healthcare professionals, dietitians, and support groups for guidance and motivation

In some cases, weight loss surgery (bariatric surgery) may be recommended for individuals with severe obesity and type 2 diabetes who have not been able to achieve significant weight loss through diet and exercise alone. Bariatric surgery can lead to rapid and sustained weight loss, improve insulin sensitivity, and even result in remission of diabetes in some cases.

Other Risk Factors such as Genetics and Age

While lifestyle factors such as diet, physical activity, and weight management play significant roles in the development and progression of type 2 diabetes, other factors such as genetics, age, and ethnicity also contribute to individual risk.

Emotional and Psychological Aspects of Diagnosis

Coping with the Emotional Impact of Diagnosis

Receiving a diagnosis of type 2 diabetes can be overwhelming and emotionally challenging for many individuals. It is normal to experience a range of emotions, including shock, denial, anger, sadness, and anxiety, upon learning about the diagnosis. Coping with the emotional impact of diabetes requires support from healthcare providers, family members, and friends, as well as self-care strategies to promote emotional well-being.

Dealing with Fear and Anxiety About the Future

Fear and anxiety about the future are common reactions to a diagnosis of type 2 diabetes, as individuals may worry about the potential complications, lifestyle changes, and long-term effects of the disease. It is essential to acknowledge these fears and address them openly with healthcare providers, who can provide information, reassurance, and support to help individuals cope with their concerns.

Seeking Support from Healthcare Providers and Loved Ones

Seeking support from healthcare providers, loved ones, and support groups can help individuals with type 2 diabetes navigate the challenges of living with a chronic illness and improve their overall quality of life. Healthcare providers can offer guidance on managing diabetes, monitoring blood sugar levels, making healthy lifestyle changes, and accessing resources and support services in the community. Family members and friends can provide emotional support, encouragement, and practical assistance with daily tasks, medication management, and meal preparation.

In conclusion, type 2 diabetes is a complex and chronic metabolic disorder that requires comprehensive management and ongoing support to achieve optimal outcomes. By understanding the basics of type 2 diabetes, including its causes, symptoms, and treatment options, individuals can take proactive steps to prevent or manage the disease effectively. Lifestyle factors such as diet, physical activity, weight management, and emotional well-being play crucial roles in diabetes prevention and control, highlighting the importance of adopting healthy habits and seeking support from healthcare providers and loved ones.

CHAPTER TWO

Foundations of Healthy Eating for Type 2 Diabetes

Proper nutrition is essential for managing type 2 diabetes effectively and reducing the risk of complications. Understanding how different foods impact blood sugar levels, balancing macronutrients in meals, and making informed food choices are fundamental aspects of a healthy eating plan for individuals with type 2 diabetes. In this section, we will explore the foundations of healthy eating for type 2 diabetes, including the role of carbohydrates, protein, and fat in blood sugar regulation, as well as strategies for reading food labels and making informed choices.

Understanding Carbohydrates and Blood Sugar

Carbohydrates are the body's primary source of energy and have the most significant impact on blood sugar levels. When carbohydrates are digested and broken down into glucose, they enter the bloodstream and cause blood sugar levels to rise. For individuals with type 2 diabetes, understanding how different types of carbohydrates affect blood glucose levels is crucial for managing their condition effectively.

Impact of Carbohydrates on Blood Glucose Levels

Carbohydrates can be categorized into two main types: simple carbohydrates and complex carbohydrates. Simple carbohydrates, such as sugar and refined grains, are quickly digested and absorbed into the bloodstream, leading to rapid spikes in blood sugar levels. In contrast, complex carbohydrates, found in whole grains, fruits, vegetables, and legumes, are digested more slowly, resulting in a gradual and steady increase in blood sugar levels.

Consuming too many simple carbohydrates can cause blood sugar levels to spike, followed by a rapid drop, which can leave individuals feeling tired, hungry, and irritable. This rollercoaster effect can be particularly problematic for individuals with type 2 diabetes, as it can make blood sugar control more challenging and increase the risk of complications over time.

Differentiating Between Simple and Complex Carbohydrates

Simple carbohydrates are found in foods such as candy, soda, pastries, white bread, and sugary cereals, while complex carbohydrates are found in foods such as whole grains, brown rice, quinoa, oats, fruits, vegetables, and legumes. Choosing complex carbohydrates over simple carbohydrates can help stabilize blood sugar levels, provide sustained energy, and promote overall health and well-being.

Importance of Carbohydrate Counting for Diabetes Management

Carbohydrate counting is a method used by individuals with type 2 diabetes to monitor their carbohydrate intake and manage their blood sugar levels effectively. By counting the grams of carbohydrates in their meals and snacks and matching them with appropriate doses of insulin or medication, individuals can achieve better control over their blood sugar levels and reduce the risk of complications.

Carbohydrate counting involves learning how to estimate the carbohydrate content of foods, reading food labels, and keeping track of carbohydrate intake throughout the day. It also requires understanding how different factors, such as portion size, food preparation methods, and meal timing, can affect blood sugar levels and insulin requirements.

Balancing Macronutrients in Meals

In addition to carbohydrates, protein and fat also play important roles in blood sugar regulation and overall health. Balancing these macronutrients in meals can help stabilize blood sugar levels, prevent hunger, and promote satiety.

Role of Protein and Fat in Blood Sugar Regulation

Protein and fat have minimal direct impact on blood sugar levels, as they are digested and absorbed more slowly than carbohydrates. However, including adequate amounts of protein and healthy fats in meals can help slow down the absorption of carbohydrates, resulting in a more gradual and steady increase in blood sugar levels.

Protein-rich foods such as lean meats, poultry, fish, eggs, tofu, and legumes can help promote feelings of fullness and satisfaction, while healthy fats such as avocado, nuts, seeds, olive oil, and fatty fish can provide essential nutrients and support overall health and well-being.

Creating Balanced Meals with Protein, Fat, and Carbohydrates

To create balanced meals that support blood sugar control and provide sustained energy, individuals with type 2 diabetes should aim to include a combination of carbohydrates, protein, and fat in each meal and snack. For example, a balanced meal might include:

- A serving of lean protein such as grilled chicken or fish

- A serving of complex carbohydrates such as brown rice or quinoa

- A serving of non-starchy vegetables such as broccoli or spinach

- A source of healthy fats such as olive oil or avocado

By incorporating a variety of nutrient-dense foods into their meals and snacks, individuals with type 2 diabetes can ensure they are getting the nutrients they need to support their overall health and well-being while managing their blood sugar levels effectively.

Tips for Portion Control and Meal Timing

In addition to balancing macronutrients, portion control and meal timing are also important considerations for individuals with type 2 diabetes. Eating regular meals and snacks spaced throughout the day can help stabilize blood sugar levels and prevent overeating. It is also essential to pay attention to portion sizes and avoid oversized portions, which can contribute to weight gain and blood sugar spikes.

Reading Food Labels and Making Informed Choices

Understanding Nutrition Labels for Sugar and Carbohydrates

Reading food labels can help individuals with type 2 diabetes make informed choices about the foods they eat and manage their carbohydrate intake effectively. When reading food labels, it is important to pay attention to the total carbohydrate content, as well as the amount of sugar and fiber per serving. Choosing foods that are lower in sugar and higher in fiber can help minimize blood sugar spikes and promote better overall health.

Identifying Hidden Sugars and Refined Carbohydrates

Many processed and packaged foods contain hidden sugars and refined carbohydrates, which can contribute to blood sugar spikes and insulin resistance. Common sources of hidden sugars include sugary beverages, flavored yogurt, breakfast cereals, sauces, condiments, and snack foods. To avoid consuming excess sugar and refined carbohydrates, it is important to read ingredient lists carefully and choose whole foods whenever possible.

Choosing Whole Foods and Healthy Ingredients

Whole foods such as fruits, vegetables, whole grains, lean proteins, and healthy fats are rich in essential nutrients, fiber, and antioxidants, making them excellent choices for individuals with type 2 diabetes. By focusing on whole foods and healthy ingredients, individuals can improve their overall diet quality, support blood sugar control, and reduce the risk of complications associated with diabetes.

In conclusion, the foundations of healthy eating for type 2 diabetes involve understanding how different foods impact blood sugar levels, balancing macronutrients in meals, and making informed choices about the foods we eat. By focusing on whole foods, choosing complex carbohydrates over simple carbohydrates, and incorporating a balance of protein, fat, and carbohydrates into meals, individuals with type 2 diabetes can achieve better blood sugar control, improve their overall health, and reduce the risk of complications associated with diabetes. Additionally, paying attention to portion control, meal timing, and reading food labels can help individuals make healthier choices and manage their diabetes effectively.

CHAPTER THREE

Practical Cooking Tips and Techniques

Cooking plays a crucial role in managing type 2 diabetes, as it allows individuals to control the ingredients they use, portion sizes, and cooking methods to support blood sugar control and overall health. In this section, we will explore practical cooking tips and techniques for individuals with type 2 diabetes, including healthy cooking methods, flavor enhancers and seasonings, and smart ingredient swaps and substitutions.

Healthy Cooking Methods for Diabetes Management

Grilling, Broiling, and Baking for Flavorful Dishes

Grilling, broiling, and baking are excellent cooking methods for individuals with type 2 diabetes, as they require minimal added fat and can help lock in flavor without contributing excess calories or carbohydrates. Grilling meats, poultry, fish, and vegetables adds a delicious smoky flavor and caramelization, while broiling and baking are great options for cooking lean proteins, such as chicken breast or fish, and vegetables with a crispy texture.

Sauteing and Stir-Frying with Minimal Oil

Sauteing and stir-frying are versatile cooking techniques that allow for quick and flavorful meals with minimal added fat. Instead of using excessive oil, opt for cooking sprays, non-stick pans, or small amounts of heart-healthy oils such as olive oil or avocado oil. By using high heat and constantly stirring ingredients, you can achieve a golden brown color and delicious flavor without excess oil.

Steaming and Poaching for Light and Nutrient-Rich Meals

Steaming and poaching are gentle cooking methods that help preserve the natural flavors, textures, and nutrients of foods without the need for added fat. Steaming vegetables, fish, and poultry locks in moisture and nutrients, while poaching lean proteins such as chicken or fish in flavorful liquids such as broth or wine creates tender and succulent dishes without excess calories or carbohydrates.

Flavor Enhancers and Seasonings

Herbs and Spices for Added Flavor Without Sodium

Herbs and spices are excellent flavor enhancers for individuals with type 2 diabetes, as they add depth and complexity to dishes without adding extra calories, carbohydrates, or sodium.

Experiment with a variety of herbs and spices such as basil, oregano, thyme, rosemary, cumin, paprika, and cinnamon to elevate the flavor of your meals and reduce the need for added salt.

Citrus Zest and Vinegars for Brightness

Citrus zest and vinegars add brightness and acidity to dishes, enhancing their flavor and balance without the need for added fat or sugar. Use fresh lemon, lime, or orange zest to add a burst of citrus flavor to salads, marinades, and sauces, or drizzle balsamic vinegar or apple cider vinegar over roasted vegetables, grilled meats, or salads for a tangy and refreshing finish.

Homemade Spice Blends and Herb Infusions

Creating homemade spice blends and herb infusions allows individuals to customize the flavor of their dishes and avoid the added sugars, preservatives, and artificial ingredients found in commercial seasoning mixes. Experiment with different combinations of herbs, spices, and aromatics to create your own unique blends, such as Italian seasoning, taco seasoning, or curry powder, to add depth and complexity to your favorite recipes.

Smart Ingredient Swaps and Substitutions

Using Whole Grain Alternatives to Refined Carbohydrates

Swapping refined carbohydrates such as white rice, pasta, and bread for whole grain alternatives can help individuals with type 2 diabetes stabilize blood sugar levels and increase their intake of fiber, vitamins, and minerals. Choose whole grain options such as brown rice, quinoa, whole wheat pasta, and whole grain bread to provide sustained energy and promote overall health and well-being.

Substituting High-Fat Ingredients with Healthier Options

Replacing high-fat ingredients such as butter, cream, and full-fat dairy with healthier alternatives can help reduce the calorie and fat content of dishes without sacrificing flavor or texture. Substitute olive oil or avocado oil for butter in cooking and baking, use low-fat or non-dairy alternatives such as Greek yogurt or almond milk in place of cream or milk, and opt for reduced-fat cheese or cheese alternatives to lower the saturated fat content of meals.

Choosing Lean Proteins and Plant-Based Alternatives

Incorporating lean proteins such as poultry, fish, tofu, and legumes into meals can help individuals with type 2 diabetes control their blood sugar levels and reduce their intake of saturated fat and cholesterol. Experiment with plant-based alternatives such as tofu, tempeh, lentils, and beans to add variety and nutrient-rich protein sources to your diet, while also reducing your environmental footprint and supporting sustainable food choices.

In conclusion, practical cooking tips and techniques can help individuals with type 2 diabetes manage their condition effectively and improve their overall health and well-being. By choosing healthy cooking methods, incorporating flavorful seasonings and spices, and making smart ingredient swaps and substitutions, individuals can enjoy delicious and nutritious meals that support blood sugar control, promote weight management, and reduce the risk of complications associated with diabetes. Experiment with different flavors, textures, and ingredients to discover new favorite recipes and create a balanced and satisfying diet that meets your individual needs and preferences.

CHAPTER FOUR

Quick and Easy Breakfast Ideas

Breakfast is often considered the most important meal of the day, especially for individuals with type 2 diabetes, as it helps kickstart metabolism, stabilize blood sugar levels, and provide energy for the day ahead. Quick and easy breakfast options that are high in fiber, protein, and nutrients can help individuals with type 2 diabetes start their day on the right foot. In this section, we will explore a variety of delicious and nutritious breakfast ideas that are perfect for busy mornings.

High-Fiber Breakfast Options

Overnight Oats with Berries and Chia Seeds

Overnight oats are a convenient and nutritious breakfast option that can be prepared in advance and customized to suit individual tastes. Simply combine rolled oats with your choice of milk (such as almond milk or soy milk), Greek yogurt, berries, and chia seeds in a mason jar or container, and refrigerate overnight. In the morning, top with additional berries, nuts, or seeds for added flavor and texture.

Whole Grain Toast with Avocado and Poached Egg

Whole grain toast topped with mashed avocado and a poached egg is a satisfying and nutrient-rich breakfast option that provides a balance of fiber, healthy fats, and protein. Toast a slice of whole grain bread, spread with mashed avocado, and top with a poached egg. Sprinkle with salt, pepper, and a dash of hot sauce for extra flavor.

Greek Yogurt Parfait with Nuts and Seeds

Greek yogurt parfaits are a delicious and filling breakfast option that can be customized with your favorite toppings. Layer Greek yogurt with fresh berries, nuts, seeds, and a drizzle of honey or maple syrup for added sweetness. This breakfast option is high in protein, calcium, and healthy fats, making it an excellent choice for individuals with type 2 diabetes.

Protein-Packed Morning Meals

Spinach and Feta Egg Muffins

Spinach and feta egg muffins are a portable and protein-packed breakfast option that can be made in advance and enjoyed throughout the week. Simply whisk together eggs, chopped spinach, crumbled feta cheese, and seasonings such as salt, pepper, and garlic powder. Pour the mixture into muffin tins and bake until set. These egg muffins can be stored in the refrigerator or freezer and reheated for a quick and convenient breakfast.

Breakfast Burrito with Turkey Sausage and Vegetables

Breakfast burritos are a hearty and satisfying breakfast option that can be customized with your favorite ingredients. Fill a whole grain tortilla with scrambled eggs, cooked turkey sausage, sautéed vegetables such as bell peppers, onions, and mushrooms, and a sprinkle of cheese. Roll up the burrito and enjoy it on the go or wrap it in foil for a portable breakfast option.

Cottage Cheese Pancakes with Berries

Cottage cheese pancakes are a low-carb and protein-rich alternative to traditional pancakes that are perfect for individuals with type 2 diabetes. Simply blend together cottage cheese, eggs, oats, and a splash of vanilla extract until smooth. Cook the pancakes on a skillet until golden brown, then top with fresh berries and a drizzle of honey or maple syrup.

Quick and Nutrient-Dense Smoothies

Green Smoothie with Spinach, Banana, and Almond Milk

Green smoothies are a refreshing and nutrient-dense breakfast option that can be made in minutes. Blend together spinach, banana, almond milk, and your choice of protein powder or nut butter until smooth. Add a handful of ice cubes for a frosty texture, and enjoy your green smoothie as a quick and convenient breakfast or snack.

Berry Blast Smoothie with Greek Yogurt and Flaxseeds

Berry blast smoothies are a delicious and antioxidant-rich breakfast option that can be customized with your favorite berries and superfoods. Blend together mixed berries, Greek yogurt, flaxseeds, and a splash of orange juice or coconut water until smooth. Add a handful of spinach or kale for an extra boost of nutrients, and enjoy your berry blast smoothie on the go.

Peanut Butter Banana Smoothie with Oats and Cinnamon

Peanut butter banana smoothies are a creamy and satisfying breakfast option that provides a balance of protein, healthy fats, and carbohydrates. Blend together ripe banana, peanut butter, oats, cinnamon, and your choice of milk until smooth. Add a drizzle of honey or maple syrup for added sweetness, and enjoy your peanut butter banana smoothie as a quick and nourishing breakfast or snack.

In conclusion, quick and easy breakfast ideas that are high in fiber, protein, and nutrients are essential for individuals with type 2 diabetes to start their day on the right foot and support blood sugar control. Whether you prefer overnight oats, egg muffins, smoothies, or breakfast burritos, there are plenty of delicious and nutritious options to choose from that can be prepared in minutes and enjoyed on the go. Experiment with different ingredients and flavors to find your favorite breakfast combinations and make healthy eating a priority every day.

CHAPTER FIVE

Simple and Satisfying Lunch Options

Lunch is an important meal that provides energy and nutrients to fuel the rest of the day. For individuals managing type 2 diabetes, choosing lunch options that are simple, satisfying, and balanced can help maintain stable blood sugar levels and support overall health. In this section, we will explore a variety of delicious and nutritious lunch ideas that are perfect for busy days.

Vibrant Salad Creations

Grilled Chicken Caesar Salad with Homemade Dressing

A Grilled Chicken Caesar Salad is a classic lunch option that is both satisfying and nutritious. Start with a base of crisp romaine lettuce, grilled chicken breast, and whole grain croutons. Top with freshly grated Parmesan cheese and a homemade Caesar dressing made with Greek yogurt, lemon juice, Dijon mustard, and garlic. This salad is packed with protein, fiber, and flavor, making it a delicious and satisfying lunch option.

Mediterranean Salad with Tuna and Olives

A Mediterranean Salad with Tuna and Olives is a vibrant and flavorful lunch option that is perfect for warmer weather. Start with a base of mixed greens, cherry tomatoes, cucumbers, red onions, and Kalamata olives. Top with canned tuna packed in water, crumbled feta cheese, and a drizzle of olive oil and balsamic vinegar. This salad is rich in heart-healthy fats, protein, and antioxidants, making it a nutritious and satisfying lunch choice.

Quinoa Salad with Roasted Vegetables and Feta

A Quinoa Salad with Roasted Vegetables and Feta is a hearty and satisfying lunch option that is packed with flavor and nutrients. Start with cooked quinoa as the base, and add roasted vegetables such as bell peppers, zucchini, and cherry tomatoes. Top with crumbled feta cheese, chopped fresh herbs, and a simple vinaigrette made with olive oil, lemon juice, and garlic. This salad is high in fiber, protein, and vitamins, making it a nutritious and filling lunch option.

Flavorful Sandwiches and Wraps

Turkey and Avocado Wrap with Whole Wheat Tortilla

A Turkey and Avocado Wrap is a delicious and portable lunch option that is perfect for on-the-go. Start with a whole wheat tortilla and layer with sliced turkey breast, mashed avocado, sliced tomatoes, and leafy greens. Roll up the wrap tightly and slice in half for easy eating. This sandwich is rich in protein, healthy fats, and fiber, making it a nutritious and satisfying lunch choice.

Veggie Hummus Sandwich on Multigrain Bread

A Veggie Hummus Sandwich is a flavorful and nutritious lunch option that is packed with plant-based protein and fiber. Start with toasted multigrain bread and spread with a generous layer of hummus. Top with thinly sliced cucumbers, bell peppers, carrots, and radishes. Add leafy greens and a sprinkle of sunflower seeds for added crunch. This sandwich is satisfying, flavorful, and easy to customize with your favorite vegetables and toppings.

Chicken Salad Lettuce Wraps with Apples and Almonds

Chicken Salad Lettuce Wraps with Apples and Almonds are a light and refreshing lunch option that is perfect for warmer weather. Start with cooked shredded chicken breast and mix with diced apples, sliced almonds, Greek yogurt, Dijon mustard, and a dash of honey. Spoon the chicken salad mixture onto large lettuce leaves and wrap tightly for a delicious and nutritious lunch option. These lettuce wraps are high in protein, fiber, and healthy fats, making them a satisfying and satisfying lunch choice.

Hearty Soups and Stews

Minestrone Soup with Beans and Vegetables

Minestrone Soup with Beans and Vegetables is a hearty and comforting lunch option that is packed with fiber, protein, and vitamins. Start with a base of vegetable broth and add diced tomatoes, carrots, celery, onions, zucchini, and cannellini beans. Season with Italian herbs such as oregano, basil, and thyme, and simmer until the vegetables are tender. Serve hot with a sprinkle of grated Parmesan cheese for added flavor.

Lentil Soup with Spinach and Tomatoes

Lentil Soup with Spinach and Tomatoes is a nutritious and satisfying lunch option that is perfect for cooler weather. Start with dried lentils and cook with diced tomatoes, onions, garlic, carrots, celery, and vegetable broth until tender. Add fresh spinach during the last few minutes of cooking and stir until wilted. Season with herbs and spices such as cumin, coriander, and smoked paprika for added flavor. This soup is high in protein, fiber, and antioxidants, making it a nutritious and filling lunch choice.

Chicken and Vegetable Stew with Herbs and Spices

Chicken and Vegetable Stew with Herbs and Spices is a comforting and satisfying lunch option that is packed with flavor and nutrients. Start with diced chicken breast and cook with onions, garlic, carrots, celery, bell peppers, and potatoes in a flavorful broth seasoned with herbs such as rosemary, thyme, and bay leaves. Simmer until the vegetables are tender and the chicken is cooked through. Serve hot with a slice of crusty whole grain bread for dipping.

In conclusion, simple and satisfying lunch options that are balanced with protein, fiber, and nutrients are essential for individuals managing type 2 diabetes to maintain stable blood sugar levels and support overall health. Whether you prefer vibrant salads, flavorful sandwiches and wraps, or hearty soups and stews, there are plenty of delicious and nutritious lunch ideas to choose from that are perfect for busy days. Experiment with different ingredients and flavors to create your own customized lunch options and make healthy eating a priority every day.

CHAPTER SIX

Nourishing Dinner Ideas

Dinner is an important meal for individuals managing type 2 diabetes, as it provides an opportunity to refuel after a busy day and support blood sugar control throughout the night. Nourishing dinner options that are balanced with lean protein, fiber-rich carbohydrates, and plenty of vegetables can help individuals with type 2 diabetes maintain stable blood sugar levels and support overall health. In this section, we will explore a variety of delicious and nutritious dinner ideas that are perfect for satisfying hunger and nourishing the body.

Lean Protein Entrees

Baked Salmon with Lemon and Dill

Baked Salmon with Lemon and Dill is a flavorful and nutritious dinner option that is rich in heart-healthy omega-3 fatty acids. Season salmon fillets with lemon juice, fresh dill, garlic, and black pepper, and bake until tender and flaky. Serve hot with a side of roasted vegetables or a mixed green salad for a balanced and satisfying meal.

Grilled Chicken Breast with Herbed Quinoa

Grilled Chicken Breast with Herbed Quinoa is a protein-packed dinner option that is perfect for warm weather. Marinate chicken breasts in a mixture of olive oil, lemon juice, garlic, and herbs such as rosemary, thyme, and oregano, then grill until cooked through. Serve hot with a side of herbed quinoa, made with cooked quinoa, chopped fresh herbs, and a squeeze of lemon juice.

Turkey Meatballs with Zucchini Noodles and Marinara Sauce

Turkey Meatballs with Zucchini Noodles and Marinara Sauce is a lighter alternative to traditional pasta dishes that is both satisfying and nutritious. Season ground turkey with garlic, onion, Italian herbs, and breadcrumbs, then roll into meatballs and bake until golden brown. Serve hot with spiralized zucchini noodles and marinara sauce for a delicious and low-carb dinner option.

Flavorful Vegetarian Mains

Eggplant Parmesan with Whole Wheat Pasta

Eggplant Parmesan with Whole Wheat Pasta is a vegetarian dinner option that is both hearty and satisfying. Slice eggplant into rounds, dip in egg wash, coat with breadcrumbs, and bake until crispy. Layer the eggplant slices with marinara sauce, mozzarella cheese, and Parmesan cheese, then bake until bubbly and golden brown. Serve hot with whole wheat pasta for a nutritious and filling meal.

Chickpea and Vegetable Curry with Brown Rice

Chickpea and Vegetable Curry with Brown Rice is a flavorful and comforting dinner option that is packed with protein and fiber.

Simmer chickpeas, vegetables such as bell peppers, carrots, and cauliflower, and coconut milk in a fragrant curry sauce made with spices such as turmeric, cumin, and coriander. Serve hot over cooked brown rice for a satisfying and nutritious meal.

Stuffed Bell Peppers with Quinoa and Black Beans

Stuffed Bell Peppers with Quinoa and Black Beans are a versatile dinner option that can be customized with your favorite ingredients. Mix cooked quinoa, black beans, diced tomatoes, corn, and spices such as chili powder, cumin, and garlic powder, then spoon into halved bell peppers. Bake until tender and golden brown, then serve hot with a dollop of Greek yogurt or avocado for added creaminess.

Comforting One-Pot Meals

Beef and Vegetable Stir-Fry with Cauliflower Rice

Beef and Vegetable Stir-Fry with Cauliflower Rice is a quick and easy dinner option that is packed with flavor and nutrients. Stir-fry thinly sliced beef, broccoli, bell peppers, carrots, and snow peas in a tangy sauce made with soy sauce, ginger, garlic, and sesame oil. Serve hot over cauliflower rice for a low-carb and satisfying meal.

Shrimp and Broccoli Alfredo with Whole Grain Pasta

Shrimp and Broccoli Alfredo with Whole Grain Pasta is a creamy and indulgent dinner option that is perfect for pasta lovers. Cook whole grain pasta according to package instructions, then toss with cooked shrimp, steamed broccoli, and a homemade Alfredo sauce made with Greek yogurt, Parmesan cheese, and garlic. Serve hot with a sprinkle of parsley and black pepper for added flavor.

Turkey Chili with Beans and Bell Peppers

Turkey Chili with Beans and Bell Peppers is a hearty and comforting dinner option that is perfect for cooler weather. Brown ground turkey in a large pot with onions, garlic, bell peppers, and spices such as chili powder, cumin, and paprika. Add diced tomatoes, kidney beans, and vegetable broth, then simmer until thick and flavorful. Serve hot with a sprinkle of shredded cheese and a dollop of Greek yogurt for added creaminess.

In conclusion, nourishing dinner ideas that are balanced with lean protein, fiber-rich carbohydrates, and plenty of vegetables are essential for individuals managing type 2 diabetes to maintain stable blood sugar levels and support overall health. Whether you prefer lean protein entrees, flavorful vegetarian mains, or comforting one-pot meals, there are plenty of delicious and nutritious dinner options to choose from that are perfect for satisfying hunger and nourishing the body. Experiment with different ingredients and flavors to create your own customized dinner options and make healthy eating a priority every day.

CHAPTER SEVEN

Sides and Snacks for Balanced Nutrition

Balanced nutrition involves not only the main meals but also the sides and snacks that complement them. For individuals managing type 2 diabetes, incorporating colorful vegetables, wholesome whole grains, and flavorful bean and legume dishes into their meals can help support blood sugar control and overall health. In this section, we will explore a variety of delicious and nutritious side dishes and snacks that are perfect for rounding out meals and satisfying hunger between meals.

Colorful Vegetable Sides

Roasted Brussels Sprouts with Balsamic Glaze

Roasted Brussels Sprouts with Balsamic Glaze are a flavorful and nutritious side dish that pairs well with a variety of main courses. Simply toss Brussels sprouts with olive oil, salt, and pepper, then roast in the oven until caramelized and tender. Drizzle with a balsamic glaze made with balsamic vinegar and honey for added sweetness and flavor.

Steamed Green Beans with Toasted Almonds

Steamed Green Beans with Toasted Almonds are a simple yet delicious side dish that is packed with fiber, vitamins, and minerals. Steam fresh green beans until crisp-tender, then toss with toasted almonds, lemon zest, and a sprinkle of salt. This side dish is light, refreshing, and perfect for adding a pop of color and flavor to any meal.

Sauteed Spinach with Garlic and Lemon

Sauteed Spinach with Garlic and Lemon is a quick and nutritious side dish that pairs well with a variety of proteins and grains. Heat olive oil in a skillet, then add minced garlic and cook until fragrant. Add fresh spinach leaves and saute until wilted, then finish with a squeeze of lemon juice and a sprinkle of salt. This side dish is packed with vitamins, minerals, and antioxidants, making it a healthy and flavorful addition to any meal.

Wholesome Whole Grain Options

Brown Rice Pilaf with Mixed Herbs

Brown Rice Pilaf with Mixed Herbs is a hearty and flavorful side dish that is perfect for adding texture and nutrition to any meal. Cook brown rice according to package instructions, then toss with chopped fresh herbs such as parsley, dill, and chives. Season with salt and pepper to taste, and serve hot as a nutritious and satisfying accompaniment to grilled meats, roasted vegetables, or sauteed tofu.

Quinoa Salad with Cucumber, Tomato, and Feta

Quinoa Salad with Cucumber, Tomato, and Feta is a light and refreshing side dish that is perfect for warmer weather. Cook quinoa according to package instructions, then toss with diced cucumber, cherry tomatoes, crumbled feta cheese, and chopped fresh herbs such as mint and basil. Drizzle with a simple vinaigrette made with olive oil, lemon juice, and garlic, and serve chilled as a nutritious and flavorful addition to any meal.

Whole Wheat Couscous with Dried Cranberries and Pecans

Whole Wheat Couscous with Dried Cranberries and Pecans is a sweet and savory side dish that is perfect for holiday gatherings or special occasions. Cook whole wheat couscous according to package instructions, then toss with dried cranberries, toasted pecans, and chopped fresh herbs such as parsley and thyme. Season with salt and pepper to taste, and serve hot as a festive and flavorful accompaniment to roasted poultry, grilled fish, or sauteed vegetables.

Flavorful Bean and Legume Dishes

Black Bean Salad with Corn and Avocado

Black Bean Salad with Corn and Avocado is a vibrant and nutritious side dish that is perfect for summer picnics or barbecues. Combine cooked black beans, corn kernels, diced avocado, red onion, bell peppers, and cilantro in a large bowl. Toss with a simple dressing made with lime juice, olive oil, garlic, and cumin, and season with salt and pepper to taste. This salad is packed with protein, fiber, and healthy fats, making it a satisfying and delicious addition to any meal.

Lentil Soup with Carrots and Celery

Lentil Soup with Carrots and Celery is a comforting and hearty side dish that is perfect for cooler weather. Cook dried lentils with diced carrots, celery, onions, and garlic in a flavorful broth seasoned with herbs such as thyme, rosemary, and bay leaves. Simmer until the lentils are tender and the vegetables are soft, then serve hot with a sprinkle of chopped fresh parsley or a dollop of Greek yogurt for added creaminess.

Chickpea and Tomato Stew with Spinach

Chickpea and Tomato Stew with Spinach is a nutritious and flavorful side dish that is perfect for busy weeknights. Simmer canned chickpeas, diced tomatoes, onion, garlic, and spices such as paprika, cumin, and coriander in a savory broth until thick and flavorful. Add fresh spinach during the last few minutes of cooking and stir until wilted. Serve hot as a hearty and satisfying accompaniment to grilled meats, roasted vegetables, or whole grain bread.

In conclusion, incorporating colorful vegetables, wholesome whole grains, and flavorful bean and legume dishes into meals can help individuals managing type 2 diabetes maintain stable blood sugar levels and support overall health. Whether enjoyed as sides with main meals or as snacks between meals, these delicious and nutritious options provide essential nutrients and satisfying flavors that make healthy eating enjoyable and sustainable. Experiment with different ingredients and flavors to create your own customized side dishes and snacks, and make balanced nutrition a priority every day.

CHAPTER EIGHT

Sweet Treats with a Healthy Twist

For individuals managing type 2 diabetes, enjoying sweet treats can still be a part of a balanced diet with some healthy modifications. By incorporating fruits, whole grains, and healthier alternatives to traditional desserts, it's possible to indulge in delicious sweets without compromising blood sugar control. In this section, we'll explore a variety of sweet treats with a healthy twist that are perfect for satisfying cravings and keeping blood sugar levels stable.

Fruity Delights and Frozen Indulgences

Mixed Berry Parfait with Greek Yogurt and Granola

A Mixed Berry Parfait with Greek Yogurt and Granola is a delicious and nutritious dessert that is perfect for satisfying sweet cravings. Layer Greek yogurt with mixed berries such as strawberries, blueberries, and raspberries, and crunchy granola for added texture. This parfait is packed with protein, fiber, and antioxidants, making it a satisfying and guilt-free treat.

Mango Sorbet with Fresh Mint

Mango Sorbet with Fresh Mint is a refreshing and light dessert option that is perfect for warmer weather. Blend ripe mangoes with a splash of orange juice and fresh mint leaves until smooth, then freeze until firm. This sorbet is naturally sweet and free of added sugars, making it a healthy and satisfying option for satisfying sweet cravings.

Pineapple and Coconut Popsicles

Pineapple and Coconut Popsicles are a tropical and refreshing dessert option that is perfect for cooling off on hot days. Blend fresh pineapple with coconut milk until smooth, then pour into popsicle molds and freeze until firm. These popsicles are naturally sweet and packed with vitamins, minerals, and electrolytes, making them a delicious and hydrating treat.

Guilt-Free Baked Goods

Banana Oatmeal Cookies with Dark Chocolate Chips

Banana Oatmeal Cookies with Dark Chocolate Chips are a wholesome and satisfying dessert option that is perfect for satisfying sweet cravings. Mash ripe bananas and mix with rolled oats, dark chocolate chips, and a pinch of cinnamon until combined. Drop spoonfuls of the dough onto a baking sheet and bake until golden brown. These cookies are naturally sweetened with bananas and packed with fiber, making them a nutritious and delicious treat.

Apple Cinnamon Baked Oatmeal Cups

Apple Cinnamon Baked Oatmeal Cups are a portable and nutritious dessert option that is perfect for enjoying on the go. Combine rolled oats with diced apples, cinnamon, nutmeg, and a touch of honey or maple syrup, then spoon into muffin tins and bake until set. These oatmeal cups are naturally sweetened with fruit and packed with fiber, making them a satisfying and wholesome treat.

Pumpkin Spice Muffins with Walnuts

Pumpkin Spice Muffins with Walnuts are a cozy and comforting dessert option that is perfect for fall. Mix pumpkin puree with whole wheat flour, pumpkin pie spice, chopped walnuts, and a touch of maple syrup until combined, then spoon into muffin tins and bake until golden brown. These muffins are rich in fiber, vitamins, and minerals, making them a nutritious and satisfying treat.

Indulgent Dessert Swaps

Greek Yogurt Cheesecake with Berry Compote

Greek Yogurt Cheesecake with Berry Compote is a creamy and indulgent dessert option that is lower in sugar and fat compared to traditional cheesecake. Mix Greek yogurt with cream cheese, honey or maple syrup, and vanilla extract until smooth, then pour into a graham cracker crust and chill until set. Serve with a homemade berry compote made with fresh or frozen berries and a touch of honey or maple syrup for added sweetness.

Avocado Chocolate Pudding with Cocoa Powder and Honey

Avocado Chocolate Pudding with Cocoa Powder and Honey is a rich and decadent dessert option that is packed with healthy fats and antioxidants. Blend ripe avocados with cocoa powder, honey or maple syrup, and a splash of almond milk until smooth and creamy, then chill until set. This pudding is naturally sweetened with fruit and free of added sugars, making it a nutritious and satisfying treat.

Coconut Milk Rice Pudding with Cinnamon and Vanilla

Coconut Milk Rice Pudding with Cinnamon and Vanilla is a creamy and aromatic dessert option that is perfect for cozy nights in. Cook rice in coconut milk with a cinnamon stick, vanilla bean, and a touch of honey or maple syrup until creamy and tender, then serve warm with a sprinkle of cinnamon and shredded coconut for added flavor and texture. This rice pudding is naturally sweetened with coconut milk and free of added sugars, making it a comforting and wholesome treat.

In conclusion, sweet treats with a healthy twist can still be enjoyed as part of a balanced diet for individuals managing type 2 diabetes. By incorporating fruits, whole grains, and healthier alternatives to traditional desserts, it's possible to indulge in delicious sweets without compromising blood sugar control. Experiment with different ingredients and flavors to create your own customized sweet treats and make healthy eating a pleasure every day.

CHAPTER NINE

Dining Out and Socializing with Diabetes

Managing diabetes doesn't mean you have to avoid dining out or socializing. With some planning and awareness, it's entirely possible to enjoy meals at restaurants and attend social gatherings while still maintaining control over your blood sugar levels and overall health. In this section, we'll discuss strategies for making healthy choices at restaurants, navigating social gatherings with ease, and enjoying special occasions without compromising your health goals.

Making Healthy Choices at Restaurants

Reviewing Menus for Nutritional Information

Before dining out, take some time to review the menu online if possible. Many restaurants now provide nutritional information alongside their menu items, which can help you make informed choices about what to order. Look for options that are lower in saturated fats, added sugars, and sodium, and higher in fiber and protein.

Choosing Grilled or Steamed Options

When selecting your meal, opt for grilled, baked, or steamed options rather than fried or heavily sauced dishes. Grilled or broiled proteins like chicken, fish, or lean cuts of meat are usually healthier choices. Also, consider ordering steamed vegetables or a side salad instead of fries or other high-carb sides.

Requesting Modifications to Meals

Don't hesitate to ask your server about making modifications to your meal to better suit your dietary needs. For example, you can request sauces and dressings on the side, ask for whole grain or brown rice instead of white rice, or substitute vegetables for pasta or potatoes. Most restaurants are happy to accommodate special requests.

Navigating Social Gatherings with Ease

Bringing a Healthy Dish to Share

If you're attending a potluck or dinner party, consider bringing a healthy dish to share with others. This ensures that there will be at least one option available that aligns with your dietary preferences and helps you avoid feeling pressured to eat foods that may not be the best choice for managing your diabetes.

Moderating Alcohol Consumption

Alcohol can affect blood sugar levels and interfere with diabetes management, so it's important to consume it in moderation. Opt for lower-sugar options like light beer or dry wines, and avoid sugary cocktails or mixed drinks. Be mindful of portion sizes, and remember to drink plenty of water to stay hydrated.

Explaining Dietary Needs to Hosts or Friends

If you're attending a gathering hosted by friends or family, don't hesitate to communicate your dietary needs to the host. They may appreciate knowing in advance if you have any specific dietary restrictions or preferences, and they may be able to accommodate your needs by offering healthier options or alternatives.

Enjoying Special Occasions without Compromising Health Goals

Selecting Wisely at Parties and Events

When faced with a buffet or a spread of appetizers at a party or event, take a moment to survey your options before diving in. Look for protein-rich foods like grilled chicken skewers or shrimp cocktail, and fill up on vegetable-based dishes like crudites with hummus or fresh fruit platters.

Sipping on Light or Low-Sugar Beverages

Instead of sugary sodas or cocktails, opt for lighter or lower-sugar beverage options like sparkling water with a splash of fruit juice, unsweetened iced tea, or infused water with fresh herbs and citrus slices. These choices can help you stay hydrated and avoid consuming excess calories and sugar.

Focusing on Socializing Rather Than Food

Finally, remember that social gatherings are about more than just the food. Focus on enjoying the company of friends and loved ones, engaging in conversation, and participating in activities or games. By shifting your focus away from food, you can still have a fulfilling and enjoyable experience without compromising your health goals.

In conclusion, dining out and socializing with diabetes is entirely manageable with some planning and awareness. By making healthy choices at restaurants, navigating social gatherings with ease, and enjoying special occasions mindfully, you can maintain control over your blood sugar levels and overall health while still participating in social activities and enjoying delicious meals with friends and family.

CHAPTER TEN

Long-Term Management and Support

Managing type 2 diabetes is a journey that requires ongoing commitment and support. Long-term management involves not only controlling blood sugar levels but also adopting healthy lifestyle habits and finding a balance that allows for enjoyment and fulfillment in everyday life. In this section, we'll explore strategies for setting realistic goals, cultivating healthy habits, and finding support for sustainable management of type 2 diabetes.

Setting Realistic Goals for Health and Wellness

Establishing Achievable Lifestyle Changes

When managing type 2 diabetes, it's important to set realistic and achievable goals for health and wellness. Instead of aiming for drastic changes all at once, focus on making small, sustainable changes to your diet, physical activity, and self-care habits. For example, start by incorporating more fruits and vegetables into your meals, or aim to take a 15-minute walk after dinner each day.

Tracking Progress and Celebrating Successes

Keep track of your progress toward your health and wellness goals by monitoring your blood sugar levels, weight, and other relevant metrics. Celebrate your successes, no matter how small they may seem, and acknowledge the effort you're putting into managing your diabetes. This positive reinforcement can help motivate you to continue making healthy choices.

Seeking Professional Guidance and Support

Don't hesitate to seek guidance and support from healthcare professionals such as your doctor, dietitian, or diabetes educator. They can provide personalized advice and resources to help you manage your diabetes effectively. Additionally, consider joining a support group or participating in diabetes education classes to connect with others who are facing similar challenges and share experiences and strategies for success.

Cultivating Healthy Habits for Sustainable Management

Incorporating Regular Exercise into Daily Routine

Regular physical activity is essential for managing type 2 diabetes and improving overall health. Aim for at least 150 minutes of moderate-intensity aerobic exercise, such as brisk walking, cycling, or swimming, each week, as well as muscle-strengthening activities on two or more days per week. Find activities you enjoy and make them a regular part of your routine.

Practicing Stress Management and Self-Care Techniques

Stress can affect blood sugar levels and overall well-being, so it's important to incorporate stress management and self-care techniques into your daily routine. This may include mindfulness meditation, deep breathing exercises, yoga, or spending time in nature. Find what works best for you and make time for self-care activities regularly.

Prioritizing Adequate Sleep and Rest

Getting enough sleep is crucial for managing diabetes and supporting overall health. Aim for 7-9 hours of quality sleep per night, and establish a consistent sleep schedule by going to bed and waking up at the same time each day. Create a relaxing bedtime routine and make your sleep environment comfortable and conducive to restful sleep.

Finding Balance and Enjoyment in Everyday Life

Embracing Variety and Flexibility in Eating Patterns

Maintaining a healthy diet doesn't mean you have to eat the same foods every day or restrict yourself from enjoying your favorite treats occasionally. Embrace variety and flexibility in your eating patterns by incorporating a wide range of nutritious foods, including fruits, vegetables, whole grains, lean proteins, and healthy fats. Allow yourself to indulge in moderation and practice mindful eating to savor each bite.

Finding Joy in Cooking and Experimenting with New Recipes

Cooking can be a fun and creative way to nourish your body and explore new flavors and cuisines. Experiment with healthy recipes and cooking techniques to discover new favorites and make mealtime enjoyable. Get friends and family involved in meal preparation to make it a social activity and share the joy of cooking together.

Connecting with Supportive Communities and Resources

Lastly, seek out supportive communities and resources to help you on your journey of managing type 2 diabetes. Whether it's online forums, social media groups, local support groups, or educational programs, connecting with others who understand your experiences can provide encouragement, motivation, and valuable insights.

In conclusion, long-term management of type 2 diabetes involves setting realistic goals, cultivating healthy habits, and finding support for sustainable lifestyle changes. By making gradual changes to your diet, physical activity, stress management, and self-care practices, you can effectively manage your diabetes and improve your overall health and well-being. Remember to celebrate your successes, seek guidance and support when needed, and find joy and balance in everyday life.

Weight Watchers (WW):

Definition:

Weight Watchers (WW) is a popular weight loss program that focuses on a balanced approach to eating and lifestyle changes. It assigns point values to foods based on their nutritional content, with the goal of promoting portion control, balanced nutrition, and sustainable weight loss. Participants are assigned a daily and weekly points allowance based on their age, weight, height, gender, and weight loss goals. They can choose from a wide variety of foods and are encouraged to make healthier choices, increase physical activity, and develop lifelong habits for success.

Ingredients:

- Lean Proteins: Chicken, turkey, fish, seafood, tofu, tempeh, lean cuts of beef or pork.

- Whole Grains: Brown rice, quinoa, oats, barley, whole wheat bread, whole grain pasta.

- Fruits: Berries, apples, oranges, bananas, mangoes, melons, etc.

- Vegetables: Leafy greens, broccoli, cauliflower, bell peppers, carrots, onions, etc.

- Healthy Fats: Avocado, nuts, seeds, olive oil.

- Low-Fat Dairy Products: Greek yogurt, cottage cheese, skim milk.

- Zero-Point Foods: Certain fruits, vegetables, lean proteins, and other foods with low calorie density.

Instructions/How to Prepare:

1. Join the Weight Watchers program to access personalized support, resources, and tools for weight loss success.

2. Attend group meetings, workshops, or virtual sessions for guidance, accountability, and motivation.

3. Calculate daily and weekly SmartPoints allowance based on individual factors and weight loss goals.

4. Track food intake and activity using the WW app or website, assigning point values to foods and staying within the allotted points allowance.

5. Make healthier food choices by selecting foods that are lower in points and higher in nutritional value, such as lean proteins, whole grains, fruits, and vegetables.

6. Incorporate zero-point foods into meals and snacks to increase satiety and reduce overall calorie intake.

7. Practice portion control and mindful eating by paying attention to serving sizes and eating slowly.

8. Increase physical activity by setting activity goals, incorporating regular exercise into daily routines, and finding activities that are enjoyable and sustainable.

9. Seek support from the WW community, including coaches, members, and online forums, for encouragement, advice, and inspiration.

10. Celebrate successes, track progress, and stay committed to making healthy lifestyle changes for long-term weight management and overall well-being.

Nutrisystem:

Definition:

Nutrisystem is a commercial weight loss program that offers pre-packaged meals and snacks delivered directly to customers' homes. The program aims to simplify weight loss by providing portion-controlled, calorie- and nutrient-balanced meals that require minimal preparation. Nutrisystem offers several plans tailored to different dietary preferences and weight loss goals, including basic, core, vegetarian, and diabetic-friendly options. The program also includes support tools such as counseling, online resources, and a mobile app to help participants track progress and stay motivated.

Ingredients:

- Pre-Packaged Meals: Breakfasts, lunches, dinners, and snacks formulated to meet specific calorie and nutritional targets.

- Variety of Foods: Nutrisystem meals and snacks include a range of options such as pasta dishes, pizzas, burgers, soups, salads, and desserts.

- Fruits and Vegetables: Participants are encouraged to supplement Nutrisystem meals with fresh fruits, vegetables, and salads for added fiber, vitamins, and minerals.

- Flex Meals: Nutrisystem offers flexibility with "flex meals," allowing participants to prepare their meals using guidelines provided by the program.

- Snacks: Nutrisystem provides snacks such as bars, shakes, and cookies to help curb hunger between meals.

Instructions/How to Prepare:

1. Choose a Nutrisystem plan based on individual weight loss goals, dietary preferences, and budget.

2. Receive pre-packaged meals and snacks delivered to your doorstep, following the Nutrisystem meal plan and eating schedule.

3. Enjoy Nutrisystem meals and snacks as directed, incorporating fresh fruits, vegetables, and salads as recommended for added nutrition and variety.

4. Supplement Nutrisystem meals with water or other non-caloric beverages to stay hydrated throughout the day.

5. Utilize support tools such as counseling, online resources, and the Nutrisystem app to track progress, access meal plans, and receive personalized guidance and support.

6. Incorporate physical activity into daily routines to complement Nutrisystem's weight loss program and promote overall health and well-being.

7. Practice portion control and mindful eating by savoring each bite and paying attention to hunger and fullness cues.

8. Monitor weight loss progress and adjust Nutrisystem meal plans as needed to achieve and maintain desired results.

9. Continue following Nutrisystem's maintenance plan and lifestyle recommendations to sustain weight loss and promote long-term success.

10. Seek support from the Nutrisystem community, including counselors, fellow participants, and online forums, for motivation, encouragement, and accountability throughout the weight loss journey.

Jenny Craig:

Definition:

Jenny Craig is a commercial weight loss program that combines pre-packaged meals and personalized coaching to help individuals achieve their weight loss goals. The program offers a variety of meal plans tailored to different dietary preferences, including standard, vegetarian, and gluten-free options. Participants receive pre-portioned meals and snacks delivered to their homes or can pick them up at Jenny Craig centers. In addition to meal delivery, Jenny Craig provides one-on-one coaching, support tools, and online resources to help clients develop healthy habits, overcome obstacles, and achieve long-term success.

Ingredients:

- Pre-Packaged Meals: Breakfasts, lunches, dinners, and snacks formulated to meet specific calorie and nutritional targets.

- Variety of Foods: Jenny Craig meals include a range of options such as pasta dishes, pizzas, burgers, soups, salads, and desserts.

- Fresh Additions: Participants are encouraged to supplement Jenny Craig meals with fresh fruits, vegetables, and dairy for added nutrition and variety.

- Snacks: Jenny Craig provides snacks such as bars, shakes, and cookies to help curb hunger between meals.

- Flexibility: Jenny Craig offers flexibility with "Your List," allowing participants to incorporate their favorite foods into their meal plans in moderation.

Instructions/How to Prepare:

1. Enroll in the Jenny Craig program and choose a meal plan based on individual weight loss goals, dietary preferences, and lifestyle.

2. Receive pre-packaged meals and snacks delivered to your home or pick them up at a Jenny Craig center, following the meal plan and eating schedule provided.

3. Enjoy Jenny Craig meals and snacks as directed, incorporating fresh fruits, vegetables, and dairy as recommended for added nutrition and variety.

4. Supplement Jenny Craig meals with water or other non-caloric beverages to stay hydrated throughout the day.

5. Schedule one-on-one coaching sessions with a Jenny Craig consultant to receive personalized support, guidance, and encouragement throughout the weight loss journey.

6. Utilize support tools such as online resources, meal planners, and the Jenny Craig app to track progress, access meal plans, and stay motivated.

7. Incorporate physical activity into daily routines to complement Jenny Craig's weight loss program and promote overall health and well-being.

8. Practice portion control and mindful eating by savoring each bite and paying attention to hunger and fullness cues.

9. Monitor weight loss progress and adjust meal plans as needed to achieve and maintain desired results.

10.   Continue following Jenny Craig's maintenance plan and lifestyle recommendations to sustain weight loss and promote long-term success.

SlimFast Diet:

Definition:

The SlimFast Diet is a popular commercial weight loss program that revolves around meal replacement shakes, bars, and snacks. It offers a structured plan designed to help individuals lose weight by replacing two meals a day with SlimFast products and enjoying one sensible meal and three low-calorie snacks. The program provides portion-controlled, calorie-controlled meals and encourages participants to follow a balanced diet, incorporating fruits, vegetables, lean proteins, and whole grains alongside

SlimFast products. Additionally, SlimFast offers support tools, online resources, and a community for motivation and accountability.

Ingredients:

- SlimFast Shakes: Meal replacement shakes available in various flavors, formulated to provide essential nutrients and promote satiety.

- SlimFast Bars: Meal replacement bars available in different flavors, offering a convenient and portable option for on-the-go nutrition.

- SlimFast Snacks: Low-calorie snacks such as snack bars, chips, and crisps designed to satisfy hunger between meals.

Instructions/How to Prepare:

1. Choose a SlimFast plan based on individual weight loss goals, dietary preferences, and lifestyle.

2. Replace two meals a day with SlimFast shakes or bars, enjoying one sensible meal and three low-calorie snacks.

3. Follow the SlimFast meal plan and eating schedule, incorporating fruits, vegetables, lean proteins, and whole grains into sensible meals and snacks.

4. Drink plenty of water throughout the day to stay hydrated and promote overall health and well-being.

5. Utilize support tools such as online resources, meal planners, and the SlimFast app to track progress, access meal plans, and stay motivated.

6. Incorporate physical activity into daily routines to complement the SlimFast weight loss program and promote overall fitness and well-being.

7. Practice portion control and mindful eating by paying attention to hunger and fullness cues and savoring each bite.

8. Monitor weight loss progress and adjust meal plans as needed to achieve and maintain desired results.

9. Continue following the SlimFast maintenance plan and lifestyle recommendations to sustain weight loss and promote long-term success.

10. Seek support from the SlimFast community, including counselors, fellow participants, and online forums, for motivation, encouragement, and accountability throughout the weight loss journey.

Volumetrics Diet:

Definition:

The Volumetrics Diet, developed by Barbara Rolls, PhD, emphasizes eating high-volume, low-calorie foods to promote satiety and weight loss. It focuses on consuming foods that are low in energy density (calories per gram) but high in volume, such as fruits, vegetables, whole grains, and lean proteins. By emphasizing foods with high water content, fiber, and nutrients, the Volumetrics Diet aims to help individuals feel full and satisfied while consuming fewer calories. The diet offers flexibility and variety, allowing participants to enjoy a wide range of foods while still achieving weight loss goals.

Ingredients:

- Fruits: Berries, apples, oranges, bananas, mangoes, melons, etc.

- Vegetables: Leafy greens, broccoli, cauliflower, bell peppers, carrots, onions, etc.

- Whole Grains: Brown rice, quinoa, oats, barley, whole wheat bread, whole grain pasta.

- Lean Proteins: Chicken, turkey, fish, seafood, tofu, tempeh, lean cuts of beef or pork.

- Healthy Fats: Avocado, nuts, seeds, olive oil.

- Low-Calorie Foods: Soups, salads, broth-based dishes, fruits, vegetables, and foods with high water content and low energy density.

Instructions/How to Prepare:

1. Familiarize yourself with the concept of energy density and how it influences food choices and portion sizes.

2. Focus on consuming foods that are low in energy density, such as fruits, vegetables, whole grains, and lean proteins, as the foundation of meals and snacks.

3. Prioritize water-rich foods like soups, salads, and broth-based dishes to increase meal volume without adding extra calories.

4. Incorporate fiber-rich foods such as fruits, vegetables, whole grains, and legumes to promote satiety and support digestive health.

5. Use portion control techniques such as measuring food portions, using smaller plates, and being mindful of serving sizes to manage calorie intake.

6. Be strategic with meal planning and food choices, opting for nutrient-dense foods that provide essential vitamins, minerals, and antioxidants.

7. Include a variety of flavors, textures, and colors in meals to enhance satisfaction and enjoyment.

8. Practice mindful eating by paying attention to hunger and fullness cues, eating slowly, and savoring each bite.

9. Stay hydrated by drinking plenty of water throughout the day, as thirst can sometimes be mistaken for hunger.

10. Monitor weight loss progress and adjust meal plans as needed to achieve and maintain desired results while incorporating lifelong habits for long-term health and well-being.

SparkPeople Diet:

Definition:

The SparkPeople Diet is an online weight loss and wellness program that offers tools, resources, and support for individuals looking to achieve their health and fitness goals. The program provides personalized meal plans, workout routines, tracking tools, and a supportive community to help participants make sustainable lifestyle changes. The SparkPeople Diet focuses on a balanced approach to nutrition, exercise, and behavior change, emphasizing portion control, mindful eating, and regular physical activity. It encourages participants to set realistic goals, track progress, and celebrate successes along the way.

Ingredients:

- Balanced Meals: SparkPeople provides personalized meal plans tailored to individual dietary preferences, calorie needs, and weight loss goals.

- Nutrient-Dense Foods: Participants are encouraged to incorporate a variety of fruits, vegetables, whole grains, lean proteins, and healthy fats into their meals and snacks.

- Portion Control: SparkPeople emphasizes portion control techniques such as measuring food portions, using smaller plates, and being mindful of serving sizes to manage calorie intake.

- Exercise Routines: SparkPeople offers workout routines and fitness videos for participants to incorporate regular physical activity into their daily routines.

- Tracking Tools: SparkPeople provides tracking tools for food intake, exercise, weight loss progress, and other health metrics to help participants stay accountable and monitor their success.

- Supportive Community: SparkPeople offers a supportive online community where participants can connect with others, share experiences, and receive encouragement and motivation.

Instructions/How to Prepare:

1. Sign up for the SparkPeople program and create a personalized profile, including information about dietary preferences, weight loss goals, and activity level.

2. Receive personalized meal plans, workout routines, and tracking tools based on individual needs and goals.

3. Follow the SparkPeople meal plan, incorporating a variety of nutrient-dense foods such as fruits, vegetables, whole grains, lean proteins, and healthy fats into meals and snacks.

4. Practice portion control by measuring food portions, using smaller plates, and being mindful of serving sizes to manage calorie intake.

5. Incorporate regular physical activity into daily routines, following SparkPeople workout routines and fitness videos or engaging in other forms of exercise that are enjoyable and sustainable.

6. Use SparkPeople tracking tools to monitor food intake, exercise, weight loss progress, and other health metrics, staying accountable and motivated along the way.

7. Engage with the SparkPeople community, connecting with others, sharing experiences, and receiving encouragement and support throughout the weight loss journey.

8. Be patient and consistent, recognizing that weight loss and lifestyle changes take time and effort, and celebrating successes along the way.

9. Adjust meal plans, workout routines, and goals as needed based on progress and feedback, staying flexible and adaptable to individual needs and preferences.

10. Embrace a lifelong commitment to health and wellness, incorporating healthy habits into daily life and continuing to strive for improvement and success.

Glycemic Load Diet:

Definition:

The Glycemic Load Diet focuses on managing blood sugar levels by selecting foods based on their glycemic load, which takes into account both the quality and quantity of carbohydrates in a serving of food. The diet aims to minimize blood sugar spikes and promote stable energy levels by emphasizing foods with a low glycemic load, such as fruits, vegetables, whole grains, lean proteins, and healthy fats. It encourages portion control, balanced meals, and mindful eating to support overall health and well-being.

Ingredients:

- Low-Glycemic Foods: Fruits, vegetables, whole grains, legumes, nuts, seeds, lean proteins, and healthy fats.

- High-Fiber Foods: Foods high in fiber such as fruits, vegetables, whole grains, legumes, nuts, and seeds can help slow the absorption of carbohydrates and promote satiety.

- Healthy Fats: Avocado, nuts, seeds, olive oil, fatty fish (salmon, mackerel, sardines) provide essential nutrients and help balance blood sugar levels.

- Lean Proteins: Chicken, turkey, fish, seafood, tofu, tempeh, lean cuts of beef or pork provide satiety and support muscle health.

- Portion-Controlled Carbohydrates: Portion control is emphasized to manage carbohydrate intake and prevent blood sugar spikes.

Instructions/How to Prepare:

1. Understand the concept of glycemic load and how it influences blood sugar levels and overall health.

2. Choose foods with a low glycemic load, such as fruits, vegetables, whole grains, legumes, nuts, seeds, lean proteins, and healthy fats, as the foundation of meals and snacks.

3. Emphasize high-fiber foods to promote satiety, stabilize blood sugar levels, and support digestive health.

4. Incorporate healthy fats into meals and snacks to balance blood sugar levels and promote feelings of fullness and satisfaction.

5. Include lean proteins in meals to provide essential nutrients, promote muscle health, and support satiety.

6. Practice portion control by measuring food portions, using smaller plates, and being mindful of serving sizes to manage carbohydrate intake.

7. Be mindful of meal timing and spacing to prevent blood sugar spikes and maintain stable energy levels throughout the day.

8. Monitor blood sugar levels regularly, especially for individuals with diabetes or insulin resistance, and adjust dietary choices as needed to achieve and maintain optimal blood sugar control.

9. Stay hydrated by drinking plenty of water throughout the day to support overall health and well-being.

10. Seek guidance from a healthcare professional or registered dietitian experienced in glycemic load and blood sugar management for personalized recommendations and support.

Low-Protein Diet:

Definition:

A low-protein diet is a dietary approach that restricts the intake of protein-rich foods, often for medical reasons. It may be prescribed for individuals with certain kidney conditions, liver disease, or metabolic disorders that impair protein metabolism. The diet typically limits high-protein foods such as meat, poultry, fish, eggs, dairy products, and legumes while allowing moderate consumption of low-protein foods such as fruits, vegetables, grains, and fats. The goal of a low-protein diet is to reduce the workload on the kidneys and liver, manage symptoms, and slow the progression of underlying medical conditions.

Ingredients:

- Low-Protein Foods: Fruits, vegetables, grains, fats, and oils are typically allowed in moderate amounts on a low-protein diet.

- Limited Protein Sources: Protein-rich foods such as meat, poultry, fish, eggs, dairy products, and legumes are restricted or limited in portion size.

- Protein-Free Foods: Certain foods may be completely avoided on a low-protein diet, especially those with high protein content.

- Fluids: Adequate hydration is important on a low-protein diet, so drinking water and other low-protein beverages is encouraged.

Instructions/How to Prepare:

1. Consult with a healthcare professional or registered dietitian to determine if a low-protein diet is appropriate for your medical condition and health needs.

2. Receive personalized guidance on the recommended daily intake of protein, as well as specific dietary restrictions and allowances.

3. Identify high-protein foods to limit or avoid, including meat, poultry, fish, eggs, dairy products, and legumes.

4. Plan meals and snacks that emphasize low-protein foods such as fruits, vegetables, grains, and fats while limiting protein-rich ingredients.

5. Use portion control techniques to manage protein intake and ensure compliance with dietary recommendations.

6. Explore alternative protein sources that are lower in protein content, such as tofu, tempeh, seitan, and certain grains and vegetables.

7. Monitor symptoms and adjust dietary choices as needed based on individual tolerance and response to the low-protein diet.

8. Stay hydrated by drinking plenty of water throughout the day, as adequate fluid intake is important for kidney function and overall health.

9. Consider working with a registered dietitian experienced in medical nutrition therapy to develop a customized meal plan and receive ongoing support and guidance.

10.   Regularly follow up with healthcare providers to assess progress, monitor kidney function, and adjust dietary recommendations as needed.

The Fast Diet (5:2 Diet):

Definition:

The Fast Diet, also known as the 5:2 Diet, is a popular intermittent fasting approach that involves alternating between regular eating days and fasting days. On fasting days, individuals restrict calorie intake to a quarter of their usual daily intake, typically around 500-600 calories for women and 600-800 calories for men. On non-fasting days, individuals eat normally without calorie restriction. The Fast Diet is believed to promote weight loss, improve metabolic health, and provide other potential health benefits by inducing a state of mild calorie restriction and metabolic adaptation.

Ingredients:

- Regular Eating Days: On non-fasting days, individuals can eat a balanced diet that includes a variety of foods such as fruits, vegetables, whole grains, lean proteins, and healthy fats.

- Fasting Days: On fasting days, individuals consume a limited number of calories, typically from low-calorie foods such as vegetables, fruits, lean proteins, and small amounts of grains and fats.

- Fluids: Adequate hydration is important on fasting days, so drinking water, herbal tea, and other non-caloric beverages is encouraged.

Instructions/How to Prepare:

1. Determine fasting days and non-fasting days based on personal preferences, lifestyle, and schedule.

2. Plan meals and snacks for non-fasting days that provide balanced nutrition and meet individual dietary preferences and calorie needs.

3. On fasting days, consume a limited number of calories, typically around 500-600 calories for women and 600-800 calories for men, spread throughout the day.

4. Choose low-calorie foods that provide satiety and essential nutrients, such as vegetables, fruits, lean proteins, and small amounts of grains and fats.

5. Practice portion control and mindful eating on both fasting and non-fasting days to manage calorie intake and support overall health and well-being.

6. Stay hydrated by drinking plenty of water throughout the day, especially on fasting days when calorie intake is restricted.

7. Consider experimenting with different fasting schedules, such as alternate-day fasting or modified fasting, to find what works best for individual preferences and goals.

8. Be patient and flexible, recognizing that intermittent fasting may take time to adapt to and may not be suitable for everyone.

9. Monitor hunger, energy levels, and overall well-being throughout the fasting period, adjusting dietary choices and fasting schedules as needed.

10. Consult with a healthcare professional or registered dietitian before starting the Fast Diet, especially if you have underlying health conditions or concerns about fasting.

The Blood Sugar Solution Diet:

Definition:

The Blood Sugar Solution Diet, developed by Dr. Mark Hyman, is a comprehensive approach to managing blood sugar levels and promoting overall health and well-being. It focuses on reducing inflammation, balancing blood sugar, and optimizing metabolism through dietary changes, lifestyle modifications, and targeted supplementation. The diet emphasizes whole, nutrient-dense foods that support stable blood sugar levels, such as non-starchy vegetables, lean proteins, healthy fats, and low-glycemic carbohydrates. It also encourages individuals to eliminate processed foods, refined sugars, artificial additives, and other inflammatory substances from their diet to reduce insulin resistance and improve metabolic function.

Ingredients:

- Whole Foods: Non-starchy vegetables, leafy greens, lean proteins, nuts, seeds, legumes, whole grains, healthy fats, and low-glycemic fruits are emphasized on The Blood Sugar Solution Diet.

- Nutrient-Dense Foods: Foods rich in essential nutrients, vitamins, minerals, and antioxidants are prioritized to support overall health and well-being.

- Elimination of Processed Foods: Processed foods, refined sugars, artificial additives, trans fats, and other inflammatory substances are eliminated or minimized to reduce inflammation and support metabolic health.

- Hydration: Adequate hydration is important on The Blood Sugar Solution Diet, so drinking water, herbal tea, and other non-caloric beverages is encouraged.

Instructions/How to Prepare:

1. Familiarize yourself with the principles of The Blood Sugar Solution Diet, including recommendations for food choices, portion sizes, meal timing, and lifestyle habits.

2. Stock your kitchen with whole, nutrient-dense foods such as non-starchy vegetables, leafy greens, lean proteins, nuts, seeds, legumes, whole grains, healthy fats, and low-glycemic fruits.

3. Plan meals and snacks that prioritize whole foods and balance macronutrients to support stable blood sugar levels and optimize metabolism.

4. Focus on eating a variety of colors, flavors, and textures in meals to ensure a diverse intake of nutrients and promote satiety and enjoyment.

5. Minimize or eliminate processed foods, refined sugars, artificial additives, trans fats, and other inflammatory substances from your diet to reduce inflammation and support metabolic health.

6. Pay attention to portion sizes and practice mindful eating by listening to hunger and fullness cues, eating slowly, and savoring each bite.

7. Stay hydrated by drinking plenty of water throughout the day to support overall health and well-being.

8. Incorporate regular physical activity into your daily routine to enhance metabolic function, support weight management, and promote overall fitness and well-being.

9. Monitor blood sugar levels regularly, especially for individuals with diabetes or insulin resistance, and adjust dietary choices as needed to achieve and maintain optimal blood sugar control.

10. Consult with a healthcare professional or registered dietitian before starting The Blood Sugar Solution Diet, especially if you have underlying health conditions or concerns about dietary changes.

CHAPTER 11

DIET FOR DIABETES

Mediterranean Diet:

Definition:

The Mediterranean diet is inspired by the traditional dietary patterns of countries bordering the Mediterranean Sea. It emphasizes whole, minimally processed foods such as fruits, vegetables, whole grains, nuts, seeds, legumes, fish, and olive oil. It limits red meat and sweets, while encouraging moderate consumption of dairy products, poultry, and eggs.

Ingredients:

- Fruits: Berries, apples, oranges, grapes, etc.

- Vegetables: Spinach, tomatoes, peppers, onions, etc.

- Whole Grains: Whole wheat bread, brown rice, quinoa, oats, etc.

- Nuts and Seeds: Almonds, walnuts, flaxseeds, chia seeds, etc.

- Legumes: Chickpeas, lentils, beans, etc.

- Fish and Seafood: Salmon, tuna, shrimp, etc.

- Olive Oil: Extra virgin olive oil for cooking and dressing.

- Herbs and Spices: Basil, oregano, garlic, cumin, etc.

Instructions/How to Prepare:

1. Base meals around plant-based foods like fruits, vegetables, whole grains, and legumes.

2. Use olive oil as the primary source of fat for cooking and dressing salads.

3. Incorporate fish and seafood into your diet regularly, aiming for at least two servings per week.

4. Enjoy moderate amounts of poultry, eggs, and dairy products, such as yogurt and cheese.

5. Limit red meat consumption to a few times per month.

6. Snack on nuts and seeds for a healthy source of fats and protein.

7. Flavor meals with herbs and spices instead of salt.

8. Drink plenty of water and enjoy a moderate amount of red wine if desired (optional).

DASH Diet (Dietary Approaches to Stop Hypertension):

Definition:

The DASH diet is specifically designed to help lower blood pressure and reduce the risk of hypertension. It emphasizes fruits, vegetables, whole grains, and lean proteins while limiting sodium, saturated fats, and sweets.

Ingredients:

- Fruits: Berries, bananas, apples, oranges, etc.

- Vegetables: Leafy greens, carrots, broccoli, bell peppers, etc.

- Whole Grains: Brown rice, whole wheat bread, quinoa, oats, barley, etc.

- Lean Proteins: Chicken breast, turkey, fish, tofu, beans, lentils, etc.

- Dairy: Low-fat or fat-free milk, yogurt, cheese, etc.

- Nuts and Seeds: Almonds, pistachios, sunflower seeds, etc.

- Healthy Fats: Olive oil, avocado, nuts, seeds, etc.

Instructions/How to Prepare:

1. Focus on incorporating plenty of fruits and vegetables into your meals and snacks.

2. Choose whole grains over refined grains whenever possible.

3. Opt for lean proteins such as poultry, fish, tofu, and legumes.

4. Limit high-fat dairy products and opt for low-fat or fat-free options.

5. Include nuts and seeds as snacks or in salads for added nutrients and healthy fats.

6. Use herbs, spices, and citrus juices to flavor foods instead of salt.

7. Avoid processed and high-sodium foods like canned soups, packaged snacks, and fast food.

8. Cook meals at home whenever possible to have better control over ingredients and portion sizes.

9. Aim to limit sweets and sugary beverages, opting for natural sweeteners like fruit when craving something sweet.

10. Stay hydrated by drinking plenty of water throughout the day.

Low-Carb Diet:

Definition:

A low-carb diet involves reducing carbohydrate intake while increasing the consumption of protein and healthy fats. This diet aims to control insulin levels, promote weight loss, and improve overall health by limiting foods high in carbohydrates such as bread, pasta, rice, and sugary snacks.

Ingredients:

- Protein Sources: Meat, poultry, fish, tofu, tempeh, eggs.

- Non-Starchy Vegetables: Leafy greens, broccoli, cauliflower, zucchini, bell peppers.

- Healthy Fats: Avocado, nuts, seeds, olive oil, coconut oil.

- Dairy: Cheese, Greek yogurt, cottage cheese (in moderation).

- Low-Carb Fruits: Berries, avocados, tomatoes, lemons, limes.

- Herbs and Spices: Basil, oregano, garlic, turmeric, cumin.

- Sweeteners (optional): Stevia, erythritol, monk fruit.

Instructions/How to Prepare:

1. Focus on whole, unprocessed foods.

2. Limit carbohydrate intake to around 20-50 grams per day, depending on individual needs and goals.

3. Include protein-rich foods in each meal to promote satiety and muscle maintenance.

4. Fill up on non-starchy vegetables to increase fiber intake and provide essential vitamins and minerals.

5. Incorporate healthy fats into your diet for energy and to keep you feeling full.

6. Be mindful of hidden carbs in sauces, condiments, and processed foods.

7. Drink plenty of water to stay hydrated and support overall health.

8. Experiment with low-carb recipes and meal prep to make adhering to the diet easier and more enjoyable.

Ketogenic Diet (Keto Diet):

Definition:

The ketogenic diet is a very low-carb, high-fat diet that forces the body to enter a state of ketosis, where it primarily burns fat for fuel instead of carbohydrates. This diet has been used for decades to treat epilepsy and has gained popularity for weight loss and improving metabolic health.

Ingredients:

- Healthy Fats: Avocado, coconut oil, olive oil, butter, ghee, fatty fish.

- Protein Sources: Meat, poultry, fish, eggs, tofu, tempeh.

- Non-Starchy Vegetables: Leafy greens, broccoli, cauliflower, zucchini, asparagus.

- Full-Fat Dairy: Cheese, heavy cream, Greek yogurt (in moderation).

- Nuts and Seeds: Macadamia nuts, almonds, chia seeds, flaxseeds.

- Low-Carb Fruits: Berries (in moderation), avocado.

- Herbs and Spices: Turmeric, ginger, cinnamon, garlic, thyme.

- Sweeteners (in moderation): Stevia, erythritol, monk fruit.

Instructions/How to Prepare:

1. Keep carbohydrate intake extremely low, typically below 20-50 grams per day to induce and maintain ketosis.

2. Consume moderate amounts of protein, as excessive protein intake can potentially hinder ketosis.

3. Base meals around healthy fats, such as avocados, olive oil, and fatty fish.

4. Incorporate non-starchy vegetables to provide essential nutrients and fiber while keeping carbohydrate intake low.

5. Be mindful of hidden carbs in foods and beverages, including sauces, dressings, and flavored beverages.

6. Stay hydrated by drinking plenty of water, as dehydration can occur more easily on a ketogenic diet.

7. Monitor ketone levels using urine strips, blood tests, or breath meters if desired, to ensure you are in ketosis.

8. Experiment with keto-friendly recipes and meal planning to maintain variety and enjoyment while following the diet.

Plant-Based Diet:

Definition:

A plant-based diet primarily consists of foods derived from plants, such as fruits, vegetables, grains, nuts, seeds, and legumes. It emphasizes whole, minimally processed foods while minimizing or eliminating animal products. The focus is on incorporating a variety of plant foods to promote health and well-being.

Ingredients:

- Fruits: Berries, apples, oranges, bananas, etc.

- Vegetables: Leafy greens, broccoli, carrots, bell peppers, etc.

- Whole Grains: Brown rice, quinoa, oats, barley, whole wheat bread, etc.

- Legumes: Chickpeas, lentils, black beans, kidney beans, etc.

- Nuts and Seeds: Almonds, walnuts, chia seeds, flaxseeds, pumpkin seeds, etc.

- Plant-Based Proteins: Tofu, tempeh, seitan, edamame, plant-based protein powders, etc.

- Healthy Fats: Avocado, olive oil, coconut oil, nuts, seeds, etc.

Instructions/How to Prepare:

1. Base meals around a variety of whole plant foods, including fruits, vegetables, whole grains, legumes, nuts, and seeds.

2. Incorporate a rainbow of colorful fruits and vegetables to ensure a diverse array of nutrients.

3. Include plant-based proteins such as tofu, tempeh, and legumes in meals to meet protein needs.

4. Choose whole grains over refined grains for added fiber and nutrients.

5. Experiment with different cooking methods, such as steaming, roasting, sautéing, and grilling, to enhance flavor and texture.

6. Use herbs, spices, and condiments to add flavor to dishes without relying on animal products.

7. Be mindful of nutrient needs, particularly vitamin B12, vitamin D, omega-3 fatty acids, iron, calcium, and zinc, and consider supplementation if necessary.

8. Stay hydrated by drinking plenty of water throughout the day.

9. Plan balanced meals and snacks to ensure adequate intake of essential nutrients.

10.	Enjoy plant-based alternatives to dairy and meat products, such as plant-based milk, cheese, yogurt, and meat substitutes, if desired.

Vegan Diet:

Definition:

A vegan diet excludes all animal products, including meat, poultry, fish, dairy, eggs, and honey. It is based entirely on plant foods and emphasizes cruelty-free living and environmental sustainability.

Ingredients:

- Fruits: Berries, apples, oranges, mangoes, etc.

- Vegetables: Spinach, kale, tomatoes, onions, mushrooms, etc.

- Whole Grains: Quinoa, brown rice, barley, whole wheat pasta, etc.

- Legumes: Chickpeas, black beans, lentils, kidney beans, etc.

- Nuts and Seeds: Almonds, cashews, sunflower seeds, chia seeds, etc.

- Plant-Based Proteins: Tofu, tempeh, seitan, soy-based meat substitutes, etc.

- Healthy Fats: Avocado, olive oil, coconut oil, nuts, seeds, etc.

- Plant-Based Dairy Alternatives: Almond milk, coconut milk, soy milk, vegan cheese, vegan yogurt, etc.

Instructions/How to Prepare:

1. Build meals around plant foods, including fruits, vegetables, whole grains, legumes, nuts, and seeds.

2. Ensure adequate protein intake by including sources such as tofu, tempeh, legumes, and plant-based meat substitutes.

3. Use plant-based milk, cheese, and yogurt alternatives in place of dairy products.

4. Experiment with vegan cooking techniques and recipes to discover new flavors and textures.

5. Pay attention to nutrient needs, especially vitamin B12, vitamin D, omega-3 fatty acids, iron, calcium, and zinc, and consider supplementation if necessary.

6. Read labels carefully to avoid hidden animal ingredients in processed foods and beverages.

7. Be mindful of cross-contamination when preparing and consuming food to prevent unintentional consumption of animal products.

8. Explore vegan-friendly restaurants and eateries or plan ahead when dining out to ensure vegan options are available.

9. Connect with vegan communities and resources for support, recipe ideas, and lifestyle tips.

10. Embrace the ethical and environmental principles of veganism beyond diet by choosing cruelty-free and

sustainable products in other areas of life, such as clothing, cosmetics, and household items.

The Insulin-Resistance Diet:

Definition:

The Insulin-Resistance Diet is a dietary approach aimed at managing insulin resistance, a condition in which cells become less responsive to the effects of insulin, leading to elevated blood sugar levels. This diet focuses on regulating blood sugar levels, improving insulin sensitivity, and promoting overall health and well-being. It emphasizes whole, nutrient-dense foods that have a minimal impact on blood sugar levels, such as non-starchy vegetables, lean proteins, healthy fats, and high-fiber carbohydrates. The Insulin-Resistance Diet also encourages regular physical activity, stress management, and lifestyle modifications to support metabolic health.

Ingredients:

- Whole Foods: Non-starchy vegetables, leafy greens, lean proteins, nuts, seeds, legumes, whole grains, healthy fats, and low-glycemic fruits are emphasized on The Insulin-Resistance Diet.

- High-Fiber Carbohydrates: Carbohydrates with a high fiber content, such as whole grains, legumes, fruits, and vegetables, are preferred to support stable blood sugar levels and promote satiety.

- Lean Proteins: Lean sources of protein, including poultry, fish, tofu, tempeh, legumes, and low-fat dairy products, are prioritized to support muscle health and metabolic function.

- Healthy Fats: Monounsaturated and polyunsaturated fats from sources such as avocados, nuts, seeds, olive oil, and fatty fish are encouraged to provide essential nutrients and support cardiovascular health.

- Low-Glycemic Foods: Foods with a low glycemic index, which have a minimal impact on blood sugar levels, are favored on The Insulin-Resistance Diet to help regulate insulin levels and prevent spikes and crashes in blood sugar.

Instructions/How to Prepare:

1. Educate yourself about insulin resistance and how dietary and lifestyle factors can influence blood sugar levels and insulin sensitivity.

2. Stock your kitchen with whole, nutrient-dense foods such as non-starchy vegetables, leafy greens, lean proteins, nuts, seeds, legumes, whole grains, healthy fats, and low-glycemic fruits.

3. Plan meals and snacks that prioritize whole foods and balance macronutrients to support stable blood sugar levels and improve insulin sensitivity.

4. Focus on eating a variety of colors, flavors, and textures in meals to ensure a diverse intake of nutrients and promote satiety and enjoyment.

5. Choose high-fiber carbohydrates such as whole grains, legumes, fruits, and vegetables to slow the absorption of sugar into the bloodstream and prevent spikes in blood sugar levels.

6. Incorporate lean sources of protein into meals and snacks to support muscle health, promote satiety, and stabilize blood sugar levels.

7. Include healthy fats from sources such as avocados, nuts, seeds, olive oil, and fatty fish to provide essential nutrients and support cardiovascular health.

8. Minimize or eliminate processed foods, refined sugars, artificial additives, trans fats, and other inflammatory substances from your diet to reduce inflammation and improve metabolic health.

9. Pay attention to portion sizes and practice mindful eating by listening to hunger and fullness cues, eating slowly, and savoring each bite.

10.   Stay hydrated by drinking plenty of water throughout the day to support overall health and well-being.

The Sugar Busters Diet:

Definition:

The Sugar Busters Diet is a low-glycemic approach to eating that aims to control blood sugar levels and promote weight loss by minimizing the consumption of high-glycemic carbohydrates and sugars. It emphasizes whole, nutrient-dense foods that have a minimal impact on blood sugar levels, such as non-starchy vegetables, lean proteins, healthy fats, and low-glycemic carbohydrates. The Sugar Busters Diet also encourages portion control, regular physical activity, and lifestyle modifications to support metabolic health and overall well-being.

Ingredients:

- Whole Foods: Non-starchy vegetables, leafy greens, lean proteins, nuts, seeds, legumes, whole grains, healthy fats, and low-glycemic fruits are emphasized on The Sugar Busters Diet.

- Low-Glycemic Carbohydrates: Carbohydrates with a low glycemic index, such as whole grains, legumes, fruits, and vegetables, are preferred to help regulate blood sugar levels and prevent spikes and crashes in blood sugar.

- Lean Proteins: Lean sources of protein, including poultry, fish, tofu, tempeh, legumes, and low-fat dairy products, are prioritized to support muscle health and metabolic function.

- Healthy Fats: Monounsaturated and polyunsaturated fats from sources such as avocados, nuts, seeds, olive oil, and fatty fish are encouraged to provide essential nutrients and support cardiovascular health.

Instructions/How to Prepare:

1. Familiarize yourself with the principles of The Sugar Busters Diet, including recommendations for food choices, portion sizes, meal timing, and lifestyle habits.

2. Stock your kitchen with whole, nutrient-dense foods such as non-starchy vegetables, leafy greens, lean proteins, nuts, seeds, legumes, whole grains, healthy fats, and low-glycemic fruits.

3. Plan meals and snacks that prioritize whole foods and balance macronutrients to support stable blood sugar levels and improve insulin sensitivity.

4. Focus on eating a variety of colors, flavors, and textures in meals to ensure a diverse intake of nutrients and promote satiety and enjoyment.

5. Choose low-glycemic carbohydrates such as whole grains, legumes, fruits, and vegetables to help regulate blood sugar levels and prevent spikes and crashes in blood sugar.

6. Incorporate lean sources of protein into meals and snacks to support muscle health, promote satiety, and stabilize blood sugar levels.

7. Include healthy fats from sources such as avocados, nuts, seeds, olive oil, and fatty fish to provide essential nutrients and support cardiovascular health.

8. Practice portion control by measuring food portions, using smaller plates, and being mindful of serving sizes to manage calorie intake and support weight loss.

9. Stay hydrated by drinking plenty of water throughout the day to support overall health and well-being.

10.   Incorporate regular physical activity into your daily routine to enhance metabolic function, support weight management, and promote overall fitness and well-being.

The Warrior Diet:

Definition:

The Warrior Diet is an intermittent fasting approach that involves extended periods of fasting followed by short eating windows.

Inspired by ancient warrior cultures, this diet encourages individuals to fast for approximately 20 hours each day and consume one large meal during a 4-hour "overeating" window in the evening. During the fasting period, individuals are encouraged to consume small amounts of raw fruits, vegetables, and non-caloric beverages to support hydration and provide minimal energy. The Warrior Diet is believed to promote fat loss, improve metabolic health, and increase mental clarity and focus by aligning eating patterns with natural circadian rhythms.

Ingredients:

- Fasting Period: During the fasting period, individuals consume small amounts of raw fruits, vegetables, and non-caloric beverages such as water, herbal tea, or black coffee.

- Overeating Window: During the overeating window, individuals consume one large meal that includes a variety of nutrient-dense foods such as lean proteins, whole grains, fruits, vegetables, healthy fats, and dairy or dairy alternatives.

Instructions/How to Prepare:

1. Determine fasting and eating windows based on personal preferences, lifestyle, and schedule.

2. Start the day with hydration by drinking water, herbal tea, or black coffee during the fasting period to support overall health and well-being.

3. Consume small amounts of raw fruits and vegetables throughout the fasting period to help manage hunger and provide essential nutrients.

4. Break the fast with a large, nutrient-dense meal during the overeating window, incorporating a variety of foods such as lean proteins, whole grains, fruits, vegetables, healthy fats, and dairy or dairy alternatives.

5. Practice mindful eating during the overeating window, focusing on hunger and fullness cues and savoring each bite of food.

6. Stay hydrated throughout the day by drinking plenty of water and other non-caloric beverages to support hydration and overall health.

7. Experiment with different meal compositions and timing strategies to find what works best for individual preferences and goals.

8. Listen to your body and adjust eating patterns as needed based on hunger, energy levels, and overall well-being.

9. Be patient and flexible, recognizing that intermittent fasting may take time to adapt to and may not be suitable for everyone.

10.   Consult with a healthcare professional or registered dietitian before starting the Warrior Diet, especially if you have underlying health conditions or concerns about fasting.

The Mayo Clinic Diet:

Definition:

The Mayo Clinic Diet is a weight loss and lifestyle program developed by the renowned Mayo Clinic. It focuses on making long-term, sustainable changes to promote healthy weight loss and improve overall health and well-being. Unlike fad diets, The Mayo Clinic Diet emphasizes practical, realistic strategies for incorporating healthy eating habits, physical activity, and positive behavior changes into daily life. The diet is divided into two phases: "Lose It!" and "Live It!" The first phase focuses on jump-starting weight loss by adopting healthy habits, while the second phase is designed to help maintain weight loss and continue making progress toward health goals.

Ingredients:

- Fruits: Berries, apples, oranges, bananas, mangoes, melons, etc.

- Vegetables: Leafy greens, broccoli, cauliflower, bell peppers, carrots, onions, etc.

- Whole Grains: Brown rice, quinoa, oats, barley, whole wheat bread, whole grain pasta.

- Lean Proteins: Chicken, turkey, fish, seafood, tofu, tempeh, lean cuts of beef or pork.

- Healthy Fats: Avocado, nuts, seeds, olive oil.

- Low-Fat Dairy Products: Greek yogurt, cottage cheese, skim milk.

Instructions/How to Prepare:

1. Set realistic weight loss and health goals based on individual preferences, needs, and medical history.

2. Adopt healthy eating habits by incorporating a variety of nutrient-rich foods such as fruits, vegetables, whole grains, lean proteins, and healthy fats into meals and snacks.

3. Focus on portion control and mindful eating by paying attention to hunger and fullness cues, eating slowly, and savoring each bite.

4. Limit or avoid processed foods, refined sugars, unhealthy fats, and excess sodium, opting for whole, minimally processed foods whenever possible.

5. Increase physical activity by setting achievable goals, incorporating regular exercise into daily routines, and finding activities that are enjoyable and sustainable.

6. Practice self-monitoring by tracking food intake, physical activity, and progress toward health goals using a journal or app.

7. Seek support from friends, family, or a weight loss group for accountability, motivation, and encouragement throughout the journey.

8. Be patient and flexible, recognizing that weight loss and lifestyle changes take time and effort, and embracing setbacks as opportunities for learning and growth.

9. Gradually transition to the "Live It!" phase of The Mayo Clinic Diet, focusing on maintaining weight loss, continuing healthy habits, and making sustainable lifestyle changes for long-term success.

10. Celebrate successes, track progress, and stay committed to making healthy choices for lifelong health and well-being.

The Flex Diet:

Definition:

The Flex Diet, developed by James Beckerman, MD, is a flexible and customizable approach to weight loss and healthy living. It emphasizes the importance of flexibility, balance, and individualization in dietary choices, exercise routines, and lifestyle habits. The diet encourages participants to "flex" their approach to eating and fitness based on personal preferences, goals, and lifestyle factors. It offers practical strategies for making healthier choices, incorporating physical activity, managing stress, and building sustainable habits for long-term success.

Ingredients:

- Fruits: Berries, apples, oranges, bananas, mangoes, melons, etc.

- Vegetables: Leafy greens, broccoli, cauliflower, bell peppers, carrots, onions, etc.

- Whole Grains: Brown rice, quinoa, oats, barley, whole wheat bread, whole grain pasta.

- Lean Proteins: Chicken, turkey, fish, seafood, tofu, tempeh, lean cuts of beef or pork.

- Healthy Fats: Avocado, nuts, seeds, olive oil.

- Low-Fat Dairy Products: Greek yogurt, cottage cheese, skim milk.

Instructions/How to Prepare:

1. Determine personal health and wellness goals, considering factors such as weight loss, fitness, energy levels, and overall well-being.

2. Evaluate current eating habits, exercise routines, and lifestyle behaviors to identify areas for improvement and opportunities for change.

3. Experiment with different dietary approaches, such as Mediterranean, plant-based, low-carb, or intermittent fasting, to find what works best for individual preferences and needs.

4. Focus on consuming a balanced and varied diet that includes a wide variety of nutrient-rich foods such as fruits, vegetables, whole grains, lean proteins, and healthy fats.

5. Practice portion control and mindful eating by listening to hunger and fullness cues, eating slowly, and savoring each bite.

6. Incorporate regular physical activity into daily routines, including cardiovascular exercise, strength training, flexibility exercises, and recreational activities that are enjoyable and sustainable.

7. Manage stress and prioritize self-care by practicing relaxation techniques, mindfulness, meditation, and other stress-reducing activities.

8. Be flexible and adaptable in making dietary and lifestyle changes, recognizing that progress may not always be linear and that setbacks are part of the journey.

9. Seek support from friends, family, or a health coach for accountability, encouragement, and motivation throughout the process.

10.   Embrace a lifelong commitment to health and wellness, continually reassessing goals, making adjustments as needed, and celebrating successes along the way.

here's a 31-day meal plan tailored from "The Type 2 Diabetes Cookbook for the Newly Diagnosed":

CHAPTER 12

31 DAY MEAL PLAN

Week 1:

Day 1:

- Breakfast: Oatmeal topped with sliced strawberries and chopped walnuts.

- Lunch: Grilled chicken salad with mixed greens, cherry tomatoes, and a vinaigrette dressing.

- Dinner: Baked salmon with roasted Brussels sprouts and quinoa.

Day 2:

- Breakfast: Greek yogurt with blueberries and a drizzle of honey.

- Lunch: Turkey and avocado wrap with whole grain tortilla.

- Dinner: Stir-fried tofu with broccoli and brown rice.

Day 3:

- Breakfast: Scrambled eggs with spinach and feta cheese.

- Lunch: Quinoa salad with cucumber, bell peppers, and lemon-tahini dressing.

- Dinner: Grilled shrimp skewers with zucchini noodles.

Day 4:

- Breakfast: Whole grain toast with mashed avocado and poached eggs.

- Lunch: Tuna salad with mixed greens and cucumber slices.

- Dinner: Baked chicken thighs with roasted sweet potatoes and green beans.

Day 5:

- Breakfast: Cottage cheese with sliced peaches and a sprinkle of cinnamon.

- Lunch: Turkey and vegetable stir-fry with a side of brown rice.

- Dinner: Baked cod with lemon and herbs, served with steamed asparagus.

Week 2:

Day 6:

- Breakfast: Smoothie with almond milk, spinach, banana, and protein powder.

- Lunch: Turkey lettuce wraps with hummus and sliced bell peppers.

- Dinner: Beef stir-fry with broccoli and cauliflower rice.

Day 7:

- Breakfast: Whole grain waffles with Greek yogurt and mixed berries.
- Lunch: Chicken Caesar salad with homemade dressing.
- Dinner: Grilled salmon with roasted cauliflower and quinoa.

Day 8:

- Breakfast: Scrambled eggs with tomatoes and cheese, served with whole grain toast.
- Lunch: Turkey and cheese sandwich on whole grain bread with lettuce and mustard.
- Dinner: Stir-fried tofu with mixed vegetables and brown rice.

Day 9:

- Breakfast: Yogurt with sliced strawberries, almonds, and a drizzle of honey.
- Lunch: Spinach and feta stuffed chicken breast.
- Dinner: Baked tilapia with steamed broccoli and quinoa.

Day 10:

- Breakfast: Chia seed pudding with almond milk, topped with sliced bananas and chopped almonds.
- Lunch: Turkey and avocado wrap with whole grain tortilla.

- Dinner: Beef chili with kidney beans, diced tomatoes, and bell peppers.

Week 3:

Day 11:

- Breakfast: Smoothie bowl with mango, pineapple, banana, and granola.

- Lunch: Chicken and vegetable kebabs with Greek salad.

- Dinner: Baked chicken breast with roasted sweet potatoes and green beans.

Day 12:

- Breakfast: Whole grain toast with almond butter and sliced apples.

- Lunch: Tuna salad with mixed greens, cherry tomatoes, and balsamic vinaigrette.

- Dinner: Grilled shrimp with quinoa and roasted Brussels sprouts.

Day 13:

- Breakfast: Greek yogurt with sliced strawberries, a sprinkle of granola, and a drizzle of honey.

- Lunch: Turkey and cheese roll-up with lettuce and mustard.

- Dinner: Stir-fried tofu with bell peppers, snap peas, and brown rice.

Day 14:

- Breakfast: Scrambled eggs with spinach and mushrooms, served with whole grain toast.

- Lunch: Caprese salad with tomatoes, mozzarella, basil, and balsamic glaze.

- Dinner: Baked salmon with steamed asparagus and quinoa.

Day 15:

- Breakfast: Cottage cheese with pineapple chunks and a sprinkle of cinnamon.

- Lunch: Turkey and vegetable stir-fry with a side of brown rice.

- Dinner: Beef stir-fry with broccoli and cauliflower rice.

Week 4:

Day 16:

- Breakfast: Smoothie with almond milk, spinach, blueberries, and protein powder.

- Lunch: Turkey lettuce wraps with hummus and sliced cucumber.

- Dinner: Grilled chicken breast with roasted sweet potatoes and green beans.

Day 17:

- Breakfast: Whole grain waffles with Greek yogurt and mixed berries.

- Lunch: Chicken Caesar salad with homemade dressing.

- Dinner: Baked cod with lemon and herbs, served with quinoa.

Day 18:

- Breakfast: Scrambled eggs with tomatoes, cheese, and spinach, served with whole grain toast.

- Lunch: Turkey and cheese sandwich on whole grain bread with lettuce and mustard.

- Dinner: Stir-fried tofu with mixed vegetables and brown rice.

Day 19:

- Breakfast: Yogurt with sliced strawberries, almonds, and a drizzle of honey.

- Lunch: Spinach and feta stuffed chicken breast.

- Dinner: Baked tilapia with steamed broccoli and quinoa.

Day 20:

- Breakfast: Chia seed pudding with almond milk, topped with sliced bananas and chopped almonds.

- Lunch: Turkey and avocado wrap with whole grain tortilla.

- Dinner: Beef chili with kidney beans, diced tomatoes, and bell peppers.

Week 5:

Day 21:

- Breakfast: Smoothie bowl with mango, pineapple, banana, and granola.

- Lunch: Chicken and vegetable kebabs with Greek salad.

- Dinner: Baked chicken breast with roasted sweet potatoes and green beans.

Day 22:

- Breakfast: Whole grain toast with almond butter and sliced apples.

- Lunch: Tuna salad with mixed greens, cherry tomatoes, and balsamic vinaigrette.

- Dinner: Grilled shrimp with quinoa and roasted Brussels sprouts.

Day 23:

- Breakfast: Greek yogurt with sliced strawberries, a sprinkle of granola, and a drizzle of honey.

- Lunch: Turkey and cheese roll-up with lettuce and mustard.

- Dinner: Stir-fried tofu with bell peppers, snap peas, and brown rice.

Day 24:

- Breakfast: Scrambled eggs with spinach and mushrooms, served with whole grain toast.

- Lunch: Caprese salad with tomatoes, mozzarella, basil, and balsamic glaze.

- Dinner: Baked salmon with steamed asparagus and quinoa.

Day 25:

- Breakfast: Cottage cheese with pineapple chunks and a sprinkle of cinnamon.

- Lunch: Turkey and vegetable stir-fry with a side of brown rice.

- Dinner: Beef stir-fry with broccoli and cauliflower rice.

Week 6:

Day 26:

- Breakfast: Smoothie with almond milk, spinach, blueberries, and protein powder.

- Lunch: Turkey lettuce wraps with hummus and sliced cucumber.

- Dinner: Grilled chicken breast with roasted sweet potatoes and green beans.

Day 27:

- Breakfast: Whole grain waffles with Greek yogurt and mixed berries.

- Lunch: Chicken Caesar salad with homemade dressing.

- Dinner: Baked cod with lemon and herbs, served with quinoa.

Day 28:

- Breakfast: Scrambled eggs with tomatoes, cheese, and spinach, served with whole grain toast.

- Lunch: Turkey and cheese sandwich on whole grain bread with lettuce and mustard.

- Dinner: Stir-fried tofu with mixed vegetables and brown rice.

Day 29:

- Breakfast: Yogurt with sliced strawberries, almonds, and a drizzle of honey.

- Lunch: Spinach and feta stuffed chicken breast.

- Dinner: Baked tilapia with steamed broccoli and quinoa.

Day 30:

- Breakfast: Chia seed pudding with almond milk, topped with sliced bananas and chopped almonds.

- Lunch: Turkey and avocado wrap with whole grain tortilla.

- Dinner: Beef chili with kidney beans, diced tomatoes, and bell peppers.

Day 31:

- Breakfast: Smoothie bowl with mango, pineapple, banana, and granola.

- Lunch: Chicken and vegetable kebabs with Greek salad.

- Dinner: Baked chicken breast with roasted cauliflower.

THE END